·THE·
Natural
Beauty
BOOK

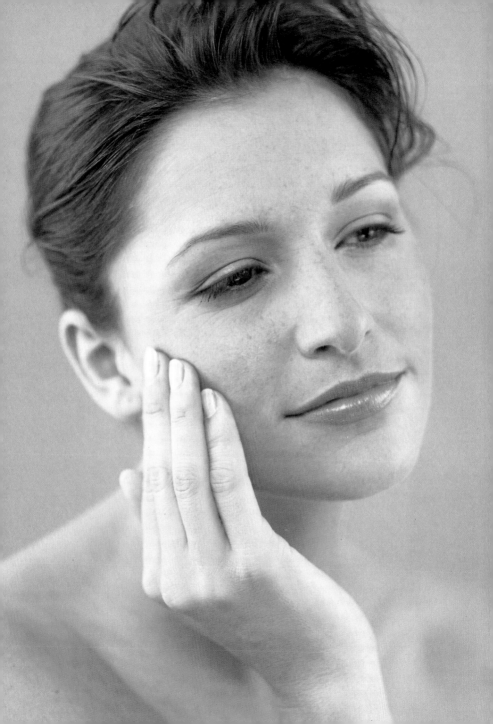

·THE·
Natural
Beauty
BOOK

SIMPLE RECIPES FOR HEALTHY SKIN, BEAUTIFUL HAIR AND VIBRANT LOOKS

JOANNA SHEEN

PHOTOGRAPHY BY STEPHEN MARWOOD AND DAVID KELLY

HEADLINE

*I would like to dedicate this book to my grandmother who, at the age of 102,
is still inspiring all the female members of the family to use pure, natural ingredients.
To Kathleen Woodger, Granny K, with love.*

Text copyright © Joanna Sheen 1997
Photographs copyright © Stephen Marwood and David Kelly 1997
This edition copyright © Eddison Sadd Editions 1997

The right of Joanna Sheen to be identified as the author of the work has been asserted
by her in accordance with the Copyright, Designs and Patents Act 1988.

First published in 1997
by HEADLINE BOOK PUBLISHING

1 3 5 7 9 10 8 6 4 2

British Library Cataloguing in Publication Data

Sheen, Joanna
 The natural beauty kit
 1. Beauty, Personal
 I. Title
 646.7

ISBN 0 7472 1956 7

AN EDDISON•SADD EDITION
Edited, designed and produced by
Eddison Sadd Editions Limited
St Chad's House, 148 King's Cross Road
London WC1X 9DH

Phototypeset in Venetian 301 BT, Centaur Festive MT Italic and Ellington MT
using QuarkXPress on Apple Macintosh
Origination by Bright Arts, Singapore
Book printed by Bath Press Colour Books, Glasgow

HEADLINE BOOK PUBLISHING
A division of Hodder Headline PLC
338 Euston Road
London NW1 3BH

CONTENTS

INTRODUCTION

Welcome to this book; I do hope you will enjoy learning more about natural cosmetics and find the whole subject as much fun and as fascinating as I do.

It must be wonderful to be a 'natural beauty'; but for most of us a little extra help is needed to embellish and take care of the looks we were born with. To do this, why not use Nature's own produce to help, rather than commercial and man-made chemical products that carry with them fears of allergies and animal testing?

Every recipe in this book has been tested by a team of people who were all sceptical about naturally produced products before they tried these; and I have incorporated their suggestions into the recipes. Cynical as they may have been at the idea of mayonnaise for hair conditioner, baking soda for the bath and bananas for sunburn, their responses came back: 'brilliant' ... 'great' ... 'perfect'! Give some of the ideas a try and you will be converted too – they really do work.

Above all, enjoy yourself and remember that laughter and love are the best natural tonics – so apply them liberally wherever possible!

Joanna Sheen

Joanna Sheen

WHY SHOULD I USE NATURAL PRODUCTS?

It is very difficult to avoid the many, many millions spent by the cosmetic industry on advertizing. Their adverts are so compelling that we all feel more glamorous if we use an expensive perfume or treat ourselves to a special French lipstick. However, if we took a trip around the laboratory or factory when they are designing and making our precious treats, we might just feel a little differently.

The number of unpleasant vats of fat and other animal products that go into many of our beauty products must look a lot less appealing seen in bulk than when they are prettily packaged and hidden away in beautiful pots and tubes.

Modern cosmetics and beauty treatments are intended to have the longest possible shelf-life. This is why preservatives are included in the recipes; otherwise the shops would have to throw away any slow-selling lines.

If, like me, you do not like the idea of unnecessary testing on animals, then by making your own beauty treatments you will know exactly what is going into your finished cream or lotion and how it was made. I have never tested any of these recipes on animals. (It did once cross my mind to rinse my spaniel with a lavender hair rinse after showering the mud, sand and sea water off her after a particularly messy walk on the beach, but she was not going to stay around long enough for me to try – she has a natural aversion to clean water!)

There is another significant reason to experiment with making your own beauty treatments – the cost. Every time we buy a pot of anti-wrinkle formula, the majority of the cost to the manufacturer will probably have been the advertizing programme that goes with it. By using home-made products with natural ingredients, you will bypass the profit made by the shops and the manufacturer, the advertizing budget and the chemical suppliers!

Now, at your fingertips, you have a world of beauty preparations. In the kitchen alone you may have enough ingredients to produce several different face masks. Instead of having to use a large pot of whichever brand of cream you have been using, treat yourself and your skin to a holiday and make a whole selection of creams and lotions to nurture a very special person!

BASIC INGREDIENTS

All the ingredients mentioned in this book are easily bought from either a supermarket or a large pharmacy. Large pharmacies are usually very helpful, especially if you explain that you are trying to make your own beauty treatments. I have had a tremendous amount of help and information from all the local pharmacists whenever I have asked for a particular ingredient.

ALMOND OIL

Almond oil is a very useful ingredient that is extracted from the kernels of ripe almonds. It is also available from pharmacies and is a basic ingredient that I could not manage without. It is not the cheapest of oils and, if economy is important, you can substitute another light oil like grapeseed oil or even sunflower oil. Just take care not to substitute baby oil as this is based on mineral oil and does not sink into the skin nearly as well. This can be of benefit for some treatments, removing make-up, for example; but for most of the skin-lubricating recipes it is important that as much moisture as possible will penetrate deep into your skin.

GLYCERINE

This comes in two forms: vegetable and animal glycerine. The glycerine produced from vegetable sources should be easy to obtain from most pharmacies. Even more readily available is animal-derived glycerine, which is a by-product of animal fat. Both types make excellent skin softeners, and you will see that many of the recipes in this book use this ingredient.

BEESWAX

Beeswax is fairly widely available as more and more people are interested in using it for many different purposes, from candle making to beauty. Granules are nice to use as they are quick and easy to measure out. However, if you have any problems getting supplies, you can also buy a block of beeswax and grate it to obtain spoonfuls. For my early experiments, I used pure beeswax candles, unrolled and melted.

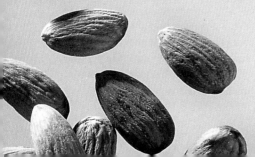

LANOLIN

Lanolin is a natural wax produced by sheep to keep rain and weather from penetrating their fleece. Although it is an animal product, sheep do not have to be harmed in any way to produce it. The lanolin is extracted from the fleece after the sheep have been sheared. For our purposes, it sinks into the skin easily and is a useful moisturizer.

Some people are allergic to lanolin, or at least to commercial products that contain it. It might be worth trying a little pure lanolin on your skin to test whether it really is the lanolin that you have the allergy to, or if the chemicals, preservatives or perfumes in that product are causing the problem.

COCOA BUTTER

Cocoa butter is available from pharmacies and is made by extracting the fat from the seeds of the cocoa tree. It melts into the skin beautifully as its melting point is the same as our body temperature.

ROSE WATER

Rose water has been a prized beauty aid and perfume for more than a thousand years. To make rose water, rose petals are infused in water and sometimes a little alcohol is added to help retain the perfume. The technique originally came from the Arabs, who used rose water very liberally to scent their surroundings and also themselves. Rose water was sprinkled on floors and carpets, and also added to washing water and even into decorative water features in courtyards and reception rooms. It is very mild and ideal for use as a gentle astringent, even on sensitive skins. However, it should be avoided during pregnancy.

BORAX

Borax is a fine, white powder made from a mineral called boron. The most popular use for borax is as a water softener, but it also acts as a mild antiseptic and helps to prolong the life of your natural cosmetics. Borax can be very soothing and is safe for all skins.

ESSENTIAL OILS

Another major set of ingredients in all sections of this book is essential oils. Once you have become familiar with their uses and benefits, I am sure you will be hooked! Essential oils are extracted from completely natural products and a single oil can contain dozens of different natural chemicals. They are extremely concentrated and most should not be used undiluted as they can cause skin irritations.

There are two ways of extracting the essential oil from a plant: steam or solvent distillation. The majority of high-quality essential oils that you buy from pharmacies, beauty shops or herbal suppliers have been extracted by steam distillation. This involves heating the plant material to very high temperatures and collecting the steam, which, on cooling, separates into essential oil and water.

However, some flower essences are collected by heating with a chemical. In this case, the oil is described as an absolute. So, if you see 'rose absolute', you know it has been extracted using the second method. It is very rare for the more expensive floral oils to be collected by the steam method. Particularly expensive oils are also sold in dilution (for example, 5 per cent dilute). This will still be strong enough for your purposes and will bring the oil within your budget.

Do make sure that you buy your essential oils from a reputable supplier and always check the labels. Only buy pure essential oils. Do not buy anything labelled 'aromatherapy oil' or 'fragrance oil' or, worst of all, 'pot-pourri fragrance oil'. It is very important to have the best product that is completely natural and will impart its many special properties to help you look healthier and happier!

I cannot stress too heavily how brilliant essential oils are and, most of all, my favourite ingredient: lavender oil. If I were only allowed one thing in my medicine cabinet, it would be this. Apart from the many beauty-related benefits that are described in this book, lavender essential oil has many medicinal uses. It is an analgesic, antiseptic, mild antibiotic, and can act as an antidepressant. It is also very safe to use, and can even be used during pregnancy.

Here are some basic oils that would be ideal to start with; you can build up your collection as you become more familiar with them.

BERGAMOT

A mild antiseptic with an uplifting citrus scent, but can irritate sensitive skin and cause discoloration if put on skin which is exposed to the sun.

GERANIUM

A lovely soft fragrance, it is an anti-depressant, aids relaxation and is mildly antiseptic. It is suitable for all skin types, unless very sensitive.

JASMINE

A very special scent, ideal for baths and all cosmetic purposes, this is an antidepressant and an aphrodisiac.

LAVENDER

This treats bites, stings, acne, dandruff, headaches and also helps to induce relaxation and sleep. You can apply it neat to your skin and it is safe to use at any time (when you are pregnant, for instance).

LEMON

Extracted from the outer peel of the lemon, this is great on its own or with floral scents. Use sparingly.

MINT

This popular scent combats stress and fatigue. Spearmint oil is very similar with milder effects.

NEROLI

A beautiful perfume made from orange flowers, this is calming, soothing and a mild aphrodisiac.

ORANGE

An uplifting citrus perfume that is excellent for dull skin and helps relieve tension and stress.

PATCHOULI

A popular perfume in the 1960s, used extensively in India, this oil helps with exhaustion and stress-related problems and is, apparently, an aphrodisiac.

ROSE ABSOLUTE OR OTTO

This favourite is also an excellent antidepressant. This is a very safe oil, but do not use when pregnant.

ROSEMARY

This strengthening, stimulating and invigorating oil has a particular affinity with the hair, and is also said to aid memory. Take care not to use when pregnant.

TEA TREE

This antiseptic and anti-bacterial oil is a powerful stimulant to the immune system. It is also an excellent treatment against dandruff.

YLANG-YLANG

A sweet, exotic fragrance which is a powerful stimulant, apparently with aphrodisiac qualities.

HERBS

Luckily, fresh herbs, and indeed growing herbs, can easily be bought from supermarkets and garden centres these days. If you are no gardener, then you may well be able to buy any of the fresh herbs you require for your beauty products. If you cannot find the herb fresh and have no way of growing them, there are many mail-order suppliers of dried herbs, some of which are listed at the back of the book (*see Useful Addresses pages 126–7*).

If you have the smallest amount of space, for example a sunny window sill or window box, then you can grow your own herbs. Better still would be a spot outside that you can cultivate as a herb patch. It is always easier to have herbs just near the back door if they are outside, as it saves trailing down the garden when it is dark or raining! If you are growing herbs indoors, then you may have a more difficult time with larger plants such as lavender and mint. These are much better suited to outdoor sites.

The easiest way to cultivate herbs is to buy a small plant from a garden centre and to follow the instructions on the label. The main herbs that you will find useful for making up your own beauty treatments are listed below. None of these varieties are particularly difficult to grow at home.

CHAMOMILE
(*Matricaria chamomilla*)

This is good for tea making as well as for eye compresses and hair treatments.

hanging in small bunches in the linen cupboard or a warm space. The flowers and leaves can be used decoratively in sachets or in infusions for your own beauty products.

LAVENDER
(*Lavandula*)

There are many uses for this wonderful plant. Lavender grows best in an outdoor site and you can gather the flowers and leaves in the summer months, then dry them by

LEMON BALM
(*Melissa*)

This herb is not difficult to grow and has leaves with a truly wonderful perfume. It can be used as an ingredient for tea or as an infusion for your beauty products.

MARIGOLD
(Calendula officinalis)

Calendula marigolds are edible and have a distinctive peppery taste that adds a special zing to salads. However, the most important use for this variety of marigold is its ability to soothe and heal skin. My grandmother has relied on a calendula cream for over 100 years now: and it certainly works!

MINT
(Mentha)

This is a fabulous herb to grow for beauty reasons and also for use in the kitchen. One word of warning: it can grow like no other plant and will soon try to take over the whole garden. So plant it in a deep tub or, alternatively, use a plastic bucket and immerse it in the flower bed — it will still attempt to escape but you will be able to tame it! Peppermint tea is excellent for calming the digestive system and as an infusion smells lovely.

PARSLEY
(Petroselinium crispum)

There are many old wives' tales about why parsley will or will not grow in your garden — for example, it only grows in a garden where the woman wears the trousers. Well, I find parsley grows beautifully in a terracotta pot by my back door but not in the flower beds, so what meaning that has I am not sure! There are many cosmetic uses for this plant, so definitely add it to the list of essential herbs.

ROSEMARY
(Rosmarinus officinalis)

This herb is fantastic for beauty purposes. Its special strength is in hair and scalp treatments. An infusion works wonders for dandruff and itchy scalps. Fresh rosemary is also excellent in bath bags for a relaxing bath.

SAGE
(Salvia officinalis)

Sage is particularly good for oilier skins, and an infusion adds shine to darker shades of hair. It is also very useful as a foot bath. This is another herb which can grow quite large, so could be another candidate for a terracotta pot.

THYME
(Thymus vulgaris)

This herb is useful for both beauty purposes and in the kitchen, so it is worth allocating a little space in your herb patch. There are many different varieties, including variegated and plain-leaved. In beauty products, it is particularly useful for hair treatments and also for tired feet as a foot bath.

STORING YOUR BEAUTY PRODUCTS

You will notice that none of the recipes in this book have any preservatives in them. There are various chemicals that will prolong the shelf-life of your potions, but I feel this is contradicting the whole point of making natural cosmetics.

The answer with natural products is to make small quantities and to keep them cool, better still, in a fridge. I will admit that my enthusiasm is such that we have a small caravan fridge in our bedroom disguised in a cupboard. This comes in very handy for chilled facial splashes, creams and lotions, not to mention the odd bottle of champagne!

Do be ruthless and throw away creams once they have started to age. Remember, you will be adding bacteria every time you dab your finger into them, and the oils and creams are an excellent breeding ground. However, if you have used properly cleaned pots in the first place, you will have a reasonable time to use your precious treatments. But if in doubt, throw it out!

One of the advantages of making your own beauty products is that you can help save a lot of packaging waste – the outer boxes, paper and general wrapping that come with commercial products. You can also very effectively recycle old packaging to make pretty jars and pots.

There are many household containers you can recycle. Small jam jars and honey pots, the small pots that mustard comes in, plastic containers from other cosmetics and medicines: all these can be reused. If you are making something as a gift, then add a little extra decoration with dried flowers or ribbons and, very importantly, a clear label and instructions on using and storing.

Do make a point of labelling everything you make, both with the contents and the date. It is very important to know when it might need discarding and it is only too easy to forget when you made it.

If you are using glass containers, like jam jars, make sure you sterilize them. This is a very simple process; just putting them through a hot dishwasher cycle is fine. However, if you do not have a dishwasher, you can also use a microwave (*see opposite*). Or, as a third alternative, jars can be sterilized by immersing them in very hot water and, if you want, you can soak them with a disinfectant tablet intended for babies' bottles.

· MICROWAVE STERILIZING INSTRUCTIONS

Experts differ on whether to put small amounts of metal into the microwave. If you are worried about this, then sterilize metal lids separately by boiling them for 5 minutes in a pan.

1. Check that the jars will fit in the microwave with their lids on.

2. Half fill the jars with cold water and cook on High until the water boils – approximately 2 minutes.

3. Remove the jars from the microwave, fill the lids of the jars with the hot water. Leave for few minutes then discard the water and drain upside down.

EQUIPMENT

You will need a few basic pieces of household equipment to make your natural beauty creams and treatments. However, there is nothing exotic that should cause you any problems; they will probably be in your kitchen already.

A bain-marie (glass bowl and a small pan that it sits
neatly on top of)
A whisk (preferably an electric hand whisk)
Measuring jug, cups and spoons
A blender
Pipette or eyedropper for the essential oils (many come with
an integral dropper)
Plenty of kitchen paper
Jars and bottles
Labels

MAKING A HERBAL INFUSION

The basic technique is used often throughout the book. For reference purposes, I have set the instructions out here. It is as easy as making a cup of black tea! Unless otherwise specified in the recipe, use:

50 g (2 oz) fresh herbs or flowers
(or 25 g/1 oz if dried)
600 ml (2¼ cups) boiling water

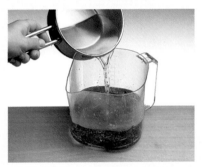

1. Add the boiling water to the herbs — a measuring jug is a convenient container.

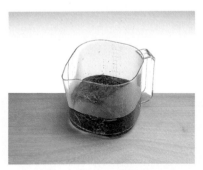

2. Leave this mixture for 30 minutes, or longer, depending on the recipe, before straining and discarding the herbs.

USING A BAIN-MARIE

When you are using delicate substances like beeswax or lanolin, they do not like to be heated directly in a pan. So, use a small pan with a few inches of water in the bottom and cover it with a glass bowl. Alternatively, melt the ingredients with the bowl standing in an oven roasting dish.

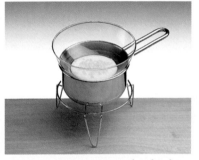

1. Melt the ingredients in a glass bowl over a pan of boiling water.

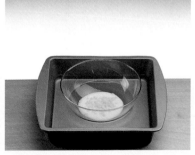

2. Alternatively, put about 5 cm (2 in) of boiling water in a roasting tin and stand the bowl in it to melt the ingredients.

BEFORE YOU BEGIN

Take your time reading through all the recipes and ideas in this book, and see which appeal or apply to you the most. There will always be some that do not appeal because you hate the smell of lavender or rose, or you may not like using face packs. It is all down to individual taste and free choice. Also, once you have found your favourites, you can multiply up the ingredients to make larger quantities, but be careful not to store them for too long. But the most important things to remember are that you will only be putting natural ingredients on your face and body, you will know exactly how they are made and will hopefully never want to revert to using only commercial products ever again!

CAUTION

Before you put any of the recipes onto your face or body in any quantity, try a small amount first on the inside of your arm and leave overnight to check that you are not allergic to any of these natural ingredients.

WEIGHTS AND MEASURES

LIQUID MEASURE (DRY IF APPROPRIATE)

1 teaspoon = 5 ml
3 teaspoons = 1 tablespoon = 15 ml
1 cup = ½ pint = 240 ml

WEIGHT

1 oz = 25 g
1 lb = 16 oz = 500 g

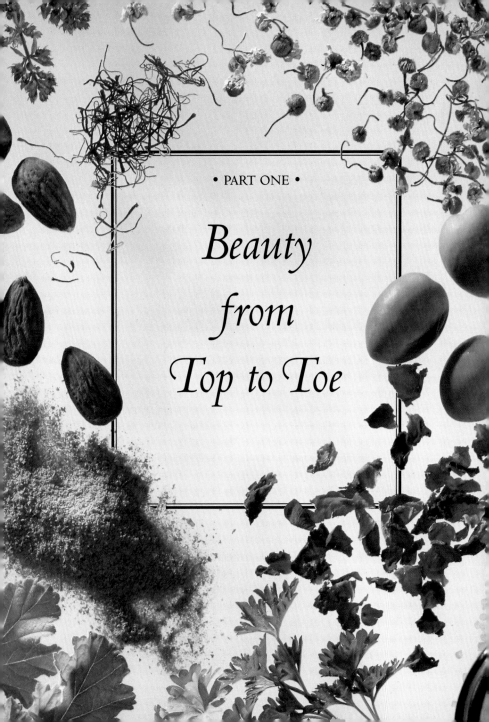

PART ONE

Beauty
from
Top to Toe

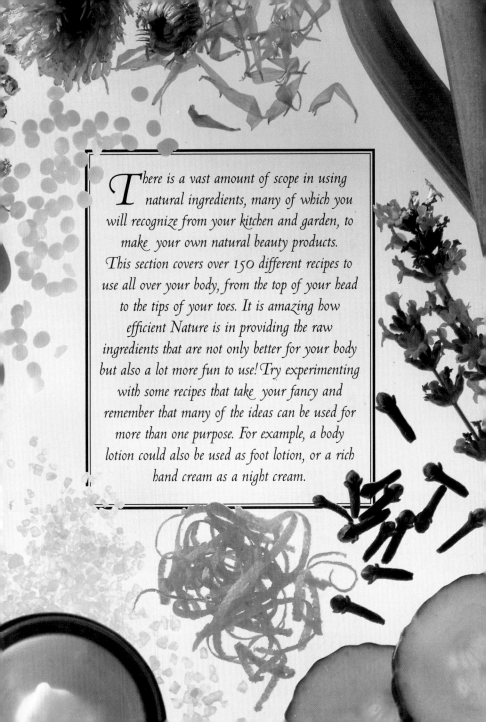

There is a vast amount of scope in using natural ingredients, many of which you will recognize from your kitchen and garden, to make your own natural beauty products. This section covers over 150 different recipes to use all over your body, from the top of your head to the tips of your toes. It is amazing how efficient Nature is in providing the raw ingredients that are not only better for your body but also a lot more fun to use! Try experimenting with some recipes that take your fancy and remember that many of the ideas can be used for more than one purpose. For example, a body lotion could also be used as foot lotion, or a rich hand cream as a night cream.

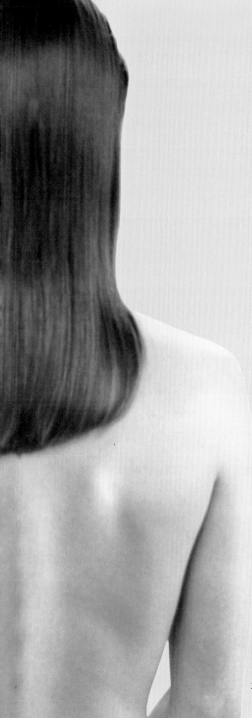

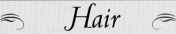

Hair

It may seem very trite to refer to your hair as 'your crowning glory', but we all know what a 'bad hair day' does to our confidence. Whether your hair is starting to thin or you have had an unfortunate experience at the hairdressers, nothing is more damaging to your self-image.

A healthy head of shiny, well-groomed hair is one of the most visible signposts to the mental and physical health of a person. If you eat well and get plenty of fresh air and exercise, take control of any potentially stressful situations in your life, and treat your hair with care, using natural products, then a stunning, glossy mane should be well within your grasp!

Your hair needs a healthy, balanced diet (*see Part Two*) with a regular intake of protein-packed foods to keep it in peak condition.

Every hair is composed of three layers. The outer layer, or cuticle, is made of the protein keratin, which protects the inner layers from bacteria and helps keep the hair moist. The second layer is called the cortex and this is where the natural colouring or pigment of your hair is made. This encloses the third layer, the medulla, which is the inner hollow core of the hair.

The outer layer of the hair has overlapping 'scales' which, when flat, protect the hair. However, when they come into contact with strong alkaline solutions — which many commercial hair products are — they stick up and allow bacteria to enter and natural moisture to be lost. This is why acidic finishing rinses, such as lemon or vinegar, can help the hair to shine by smoothing down the scales.

BASIC HAIR-CARE ROUTINE

Wash your hair as often as you feel necessary. There is no need to hold back from washing it daily if it needs to be washed, so long as you use a gentle shampoo. You should always condition your hair after washing it, and find the time once a week to give your hair a deep-conditioning treatment (*see pages 22–3, Preconditioners*).

If you can organize some time when you could leave your hair to dry naturally rather than using a hair dryer, so much the better. Its fierce heat does nothing to improve the condition or look of your hair. Likewise, too much styling with hot rollers or curling tongs can only damage your hair in the long term, and even the short term. Try to be as kind as possible to your hair and hold back on heat and hairspray whenever you can.

If you have any specific hair problems, such as dandruff, then choose one of the treatments recommended to keep it at bay. This will mean frequent washing and scrupulous care of your hairbrushes and combs, which many people leave unwashed for weeks on end. When you spend time deep conditioning your hair, soak your hairbrushes and combs in a mild disinfectant or just hot soapy water and then rinse them well.

You must be patient with all natural remedies; they may not work at the same pace as instant chemical cures. Superficial treatments, however, like the natural conditioning ideas and finishing rinses, should make an obvious difference straight away. So give some of the ideas a go. You may feel silly using mayonnaise, on your hair, but who looks silliest at the end of the day when you have beautiful, healthy hair and spend a lot less on hair products than your friends?

PRECONDITIONERS

Conditioning is a very important part of the hair-washing process. As we increasingly damage our hair by using hot dryers, rollers, curling tongs and other such gadgets, conditioners are one of the best ways to help your hair fight back. There are several possibilities for conditioning hair: you can precondition it, before you shampoo; condition after shampooing; or put an extra dressing on your hair once it is dry if it is still frizzy and flyaway *(see pages 26–7)*.

If you have very brittle hair or are trying to cope with some split ends (it is really better to have them cut off) then preconditioning is ideal. The simplest way to precondition hair is to use an olive oil massage. Warm about ¼ cup olive oil by standing it in a bowl of boiling water. Allow the olive oil to get quite hot, then gently massage it into your dry hair. Cover your hair with a towel or a plastic shower cap and leave the oil to sink in for an hour or so. If you simply do not have an hour to spare, then leaving it for even 15 minutes will make a difference. Then wash your hair in the usual way, shampooing twice.

Natural Protein Conditioner
—— for normal to dry hair ——

1 egg yolk
150g (5 oz) plain bio yoghurt

This is an excellent way to add gloss to dull, lifeless hair, and costs very little. Mix the two ingredients together and massage into your hair. Leave on for 10 minutes and then rinse off, using tepid or cool water. Then wash your hair as usual. This mixture can be used after shampooing if you prefer.

Mayonnaise Preconditioner
—— for normal to dry hair ——

Ladling teaspoons of mayonnaise onto the hair caused gales of laughter the first time we tried it but it certainly did work!

Use either home-made mayonnaise or a good-quality brand. The best type to buy is that sold in a container with a nozzle, so that you can squirt it straight onto your head, making it fractionally less messy. Rub the mayonnaise through your hair and leave on under a shower cap for about 30 minutes before rinsing thoroughly. Then wash as usual.

Parsley Juice Preconditioner
—— for all hair types ——

3 cups fresh, chopped parsley
120 ml (½ cup) boiling water

This treatment conditions the hair and helps to balance the sebaceous glands. It heals any scalp problems and boosts slow-growing hair.

Infuse about quarter of the parsley in the boiling water for 30 minutes. Then put the whole infusion, leaves and liquid, together with the rest of the parsley into a blender or food processor. Blend the mixture into a runny paste. If necessary, add a little more of either ingredient to correct the consistency. Then massage it well into your hair. Leave it on your scalp and hair for an hour or so to do its work. It is easiest to wear a shower cap while you have got it on your hair, as it does look a little strange! Then rinse and wash your hair as usual.

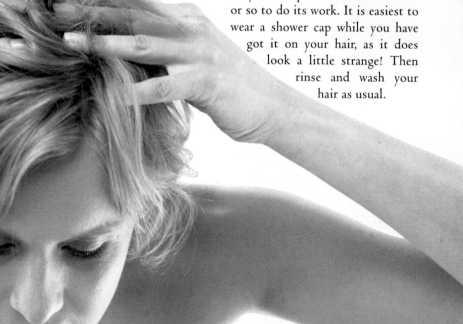

SHAMPOOS

The easiest way to impart the benefits that various herbs can give to your hair is to use the plainest, mildest, natural shampoo, choosing the best quality you can afford. You can then add extra ingredients such as herbal extracts or fragrance at home. The resulting shampoo will be gentle, but will have strong herbal properties that will boost your hair's condition and looks.

Although there are many concoctions that I could recommend as herbal shampoos made without the addition of any commercial soap product, I find it easier to use one of these basic formulas and then to concentrate on making home-produced conditioners, tonics and more unusual treatments.

The following are the basic shampoo formulas that I would recommend for the differing hair types you may have. Follow the same procedure for each recipe, mixing the oils into the bottle.

METHOD

Carefully drop the essential oils into the shampoo bottle. Replace the cap and then shake thoroughly until they are all blended with the shampoo.

Gentle Herb Shampoo
—— for normal hair ——

100 ml (7 tablespoons) mild, unscented shampoo
6 drops geranium essential oil
4 drops lemon essential oil
2 drops parsley essential oil

Lemon and Herb Shampoo
—— for oily hair ——

100 ml (7 tablespoons) mild, unscented shampoo
6 drops lemon essential oil
4 drops basil essential oil
2 drops rosemary essential oil

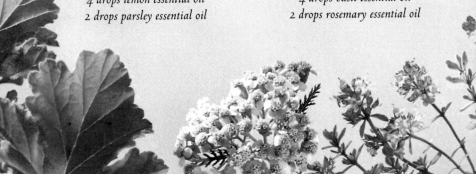

Lavender Shampoo
—— for dry hair ——

100 ml (7 tablespoons) mild, unscented
shampoo
6 drops lavender essential oil
4 drops geranium essential oil
2 drops yarrow essential oil

Chamomile and Thyme Shampoo
—— for damaged hair ——

100 ml (7 tablespoons) mild, unscented
shampoo
6 drops chamomile essential oil
4 drops lavender essential oil
2 drops thyme essential oil

Rosemary and Lime Shampoo
—— to treat dandruff ——

100 ml (7 tablespoons) mild, unscented
shampoo
6 drops rosemary essential oil
4 drops lime essential oil
2 drops sage essential oil

Egg Shampoo
—— for all hair types ——

Alternatively, if you want to be completely radical, then have a go at washing your hair with an egg.

Beat the egg slightly to blend the white and the yolk and rub it gently into wet hair. Leave the egg on for 5–10 minutes to let it clean the hair and rinse off very thoroughly. Please note that if you rinse your hair with water that is too hot you will cook the egg, which feels very unpleasant!

This treatment should leave your hair clean and shiny. Apparently it was used when no shampoo was available when my grandmother was a girl. Fortunately, they had hens – so plenty of eggs! I have to be honest and say that I prefer the herbal mixtures, but you might like to experiment.

POST-SHAMPOO CONDITIONERS

This is the point when most of us choose to condition our hair. There are many natural ingredients that can do wonders for the hair. Another advantage in making up these concoctions at home is that you will know exactly what you are using.

Avocado Conditioner
— for all hair types —

1 small or ½ large avocado
2 egg yolks
5 ml (1 teaspoon) wheatgerm or avocado oil
3 drops parsley essential oil

Apart from making you feel a little foolish, since it gives the appearance of having dunked your head in a bowl of guacamole, this treatment gives your hair a soft and shiny finish.

Scoop the flesh out of the avocado and place in a small mixing bowl with the egg yolks. Using a fork, mash the two ingredients together. Then add the wheatgerm or avocado oil and the drops of essential oil, and blend thoroughly.

Using your hands, massage the conditioner into your hair and scalp, making sure it is well covered. Wrap your hair in kitchen foil and relax for about 15–20 minutes. Then rinse your hair with plenty of water and dry as usual.

Lavender Conditioner
— for normal hair —

Make a strong infusion of lavender (*see page 16*). Take a small amount of the infusion and mix this with a few drops of lavender essential oil. This is a great conditioner for normal hair. The smell of the lavender is really wonderful and it works well to enhance the sheen, strength and body of your hair.

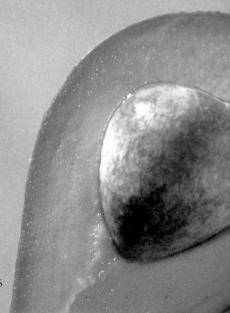

FINISHING CONDITIONERS

The third conditioning option, after preconditioners and post-shampoo conditioners, is to place a little conditioning dressing on hair that has been washed and dried. This reduces static and will help with flyaway hair.

Cream Dressing
for flyaway hair

The easiest way to control static, flyaway hair is to use a very small amount of a good non-greasy hand cream *(see page 84)*. Place a small amount of cream on your palm and rub the two palms together, then smooth them lightly over the frizziest parts of your hair.

Bay, Rum and Lavender Dressing
— for dry or damaged hair —

50 ml (10 teaspoons) rum
28 ml (2 tablespoons) water
2 ml glycerine (optional)
2 ml (40 drops) lavender essential oil
5 drops West Indian bay essential oil

You can use the small end of a child's medicine spoon to measure the glycerine; this is 2.5 ml, so use a scant measure. Mix all the ingredients together well. This mixture should be used sparingly and applied only where your hair needs taming as it may be too greasy for the normal areas of your hair.

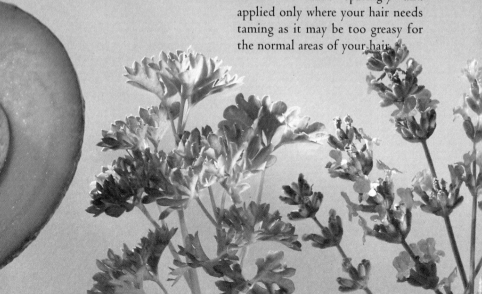

HAIR TONICS

Hair tonics are not something you often see amongst commercial hair-care products. They are a special hair treatment which can be applied as a finishing rinse. These tonics or rinses will help make hair shinier, have more body and generally look healthier. Think of it as an extra dose of help, whether your hair is in good, bad or indifferent condition.

There are various herbs and oils that are particularly useful for your hair and you will find some varieties that will crop up again and again in this chapter. Rosemary has long been a great hair improver, the same applies to lavender, nettle and lemon. We are all used to seeing them mentioned on bottles of commercial shampoo, but now you can learn to make these herbs really work for you. Start using the parts of the plants that will help your hair rather than relying on the fragrance alone (which may well be all that is used in some of the cheaper commercial brands).

There are several ways to use herbs on your hair. They can be included at the shampoo stage (*see pages 24–5*) or the conditioning stage (*see pages 22–3 and 26–7*). But one of the most effective ways of letting natural ingredients loose on your hair is to use them in a finishing rinse or tonic, after shampooing and conditioning your hair.

METHOD

To make up the hair tonic, or finishing rinse, simply infuse the herbs for about an hour (*see page 16*). Then add the essential oil, and any other ingredients included in the recipe, to the cooled infusion.

Use the tonic after you have finished any other treatments on your hair, such as shampooing and conditioning. Stand over a large bowl or hand basin, with the plug in, and pour the mixture over your hair. Recycle as much of the liquid as possible with a cup and pour it over your head again to get as much as possible into your hair. Then gently rub your scalp with mild massage movements (*see also Scalp Massage, page 99*). Finally, use a little cool water to lightly rinse off the tonic. Do not blast the mixture out by using a power shower head or something similar; the idea is that the treatment will continue working on your hair until the next time you come to wash it.

Parsley Tonic
—— for all hair types ——

*1¼ cups fresh parsley (or 2 tablespoons
if dried)
500 ml (2 cups) boiling water
2 drops parsley essential oil*

Another herb that helps all types of
hair is parsley. Some people claim
that it can improve the rate that
hair grows, and it definitely makes
hair lovely and shiny.

Rosemary Herbal Finishing Rinse
—— for all hair types ——

*2 tablespoons chopped fresh rosemary
leaves (or 1 tablespoon if dried)
300 ml (1¼ cups) boiling water
2 drops rosemary essential oil*

Chamomile and Lemon Tonic
—— for fair hair ——

*⅔ cup chamomile flowers
500 ml (2 cups) boiling water
juice from 1 lemon
2 drops lemon essential oil*

STRENGTHENING DAMAGED HAIR

Once hair has been damaged, either by over-perming or colouring, bleaching or heat, there is no way of turning it back into soft, shiny, top-condition locks. Constantly bombarding your hair with chemicals will weaken and destroy it. Try to go without hairsprays and mousses once in a while to give your hair a chance to breathe.

Keep the use of all heated hair appliances to a minimum as they damage the cuticle, leaving hair dry and brittle. If possible, try and let your hair dry naturally for a change. On a warm day, try drying your hair outside in a sunny spot. However, do not dry your hair in fierce mid-day blasts of sunshine in hotter climates. Choose a shady spot and shake your head well to throw off some of the water, rather like a dog! Towel dry to get a little more moisture out and then gently shake your hair with your fingers to dry it.

It is especially important to keep your hairdressing accessories, such as brushes and combs, spotlessly clean. Wash them well once a week (*see page 21, Basic Hair-care Routine*).

Damaged hair can be helped by applying some of the intensive conditioners, like the olive oil massage and the mayonnaise preconditioner (*see pages 22–3*). You can also try using a greasy treatment of this kind by applying the oil to the damaged hair only (not rubbing it into your scalp) and then leaving it on overnight, remembering to sleep in a plastic shower cap. This may help the hair to absorb lots of oil.

Another way to help damaged hair is to try to handle it and generally pull it about as little as possible. So wear long, damaged hair loosely tied back and stop fiddling with it, and leave shorter, damaged hair alone as well. Constant brushing and fiddling will only further aggravate weak hair.

Of course, hair does regrow, although it can seem to take forever. A normal growth rate is about 12 mm (½ in) per month and hair lives for between three and six years. So, although having split ends or badly over-bleached hair cut off is by far the best treatment for it, it is sometimes a drastic step that no one can face taking. If that is the case, then keep having the damaged hair cut every six weeks or so and gradually you will see it being replaced with healthy, new hair growth.

HELPING AGAINST HAIR LOSS

When men start to lose their hair, it can lead to immense loss of confidence in their appearance. Unfortunately, as yet, there are no easy answers to male baldness and, to a certain extent, it is accepted, even admired, in society. However, if a woman begins to lose her hair, the same acceptance does not always apply. Female hair loss, wrongly, carries with it a social stigma.

A normal, healthy head of hair consists of between 90 and 140 thousand hair follicles. We usually lose about 100 hairs a day, which goes virtually unnoticed. However, problems can arise when you find more and more hair coming away as you brush it each morning.

The first thing to do is to see your family doctor to check there is nothing wrong with you. Possible causes are stress, menopause, postnatal hormone imbalance and dietary problems. In many of these cases, the hair will grow back with the right encouragement.

The next step is to make sure your diet is good. In particular, check you are eating enough protein and vitamin B. Sulphur is another ingredient that helps produce thick, healthy hair, and can be found in several natural sources, including onions, garlic and vegetables of the cabbage family. One folk remedy for falling hair is to liquidize a raw onion, rub it all over your scalp and leave overnight. This may stimulate hair into making a reappearance, but friends may disappear at an even faster rate! The nettle treatment below is less offensive.

Nettle Tonic

2 large handfuls fresh nettles (or 1 handful if dried)
500 ml (2 cups) boiling water
150 ml (⅔ cup) cider vinegar

This tonic can help falling hair and also scalp problems like dandruff or general flakiness and itching.

Place the nettles in a pan and cover with the boiling water, bring back to the boil and then switch off the heat and leave to infuse for 3–4 hours. Strain off the liquid, add the vinegar to it, and bottle.

Massage this lotion into your scalp both night and morning. As an added treatment, use the tonic diluted with equal quantities of water as a final rinse when shampooing your hair.

ANTI-DANDRUFF TREATMENTS

Dandruff is a problem that besets many of us from time to time and some people have a constant battle against it. It is a hugely irritating condition which looks unsightly and can linger on and on. Do remember that nothing will prevent dandruff better than eating a good, balanced diet and skipping those chocolates, cakes and fatty foods! Read Part Two of this book and try to put some of the dietary suggestions into practice as well as using some of these anti-dandruff treatments.

Lavender Dandruff Treatment

lavender essential oil

One of the best remedies I have found for dandruff is to apply neat lavender essential oil, on cotton wool, directly to your scalp. Blot as much of the irritated area as possible with the oil and leave on overnight. The lavender oil seems to invigorate the scalp and the anti-bacterial properties of the oil kill off any local problems.

Tea Tree Shampoo

tea tree essential oil

Tea tree oil also helps itchy scalps and can be added to your normal shampoo. Mixing one drop with your shampoo as you apply it will clean your hair and clear your scalp. Also the Nettle Tonic (*see page 31*) is a strong remedy.

Rosemary and Lavender Dandruff Treatment

1 large handful (about 2½ cups) rosemary leaves
4 drops rosemary essential oil
4 drops lavender essential oil

This is excellent for preventing dandruff if you have a tendency to occasional bouts of it.

Put the rosemary in a small pan and cover with water. Simmer away gently for about 15 minutes. Strain the liquid into a bottle and add the essential oils.

Before using, shake the mixture well to make sure the oils and rosemary infusion are well mixed.

Wash your hair with a mild herbal shampoo regularly (daily if necessary) and then rinse with this lotion. Leave it on your hair for 3–4 minutes and then rinse lightly with tepid water.

SETTING LOTIONS AND HAIR LACQUERS

M any of us spend a small fortune on gels, lotions and potions to fix our hair into position. In many cases, we use aerosols that are probably not doing the ozone layer much good either. Here are some very old-fashioned but amazingly efficient alternatives – do not knock them until you have tried them!

Lemon Setting Lotion and Lacquer

Juice of 1 lemon

This was standard procedure in my grandmother's household as there were no mousses 100 years ago!

Squeeze and strain the juice from the lemon, then paint it on to each section of hair as you put the rollers in. Dry your hair as normal. When you take the rollers out, the lemon juice will make the hair feel a bit hard but once brushed through it feels soft and has a good shine.

You can also use lemon juice as a hair lacquer. Just spray it from a pump-action bottle and it soon dries. Adding ½ teaspoon of vodka will preserve the juice for a bit longer.

Beer Setting Lotion

Dark ale or bitter

This is the easiest of all setting lotions: simply wet your hair with some beer, preferably a dark ale or bitter, as these work best. This will give added body and help the curls to stay in.

Simple Setting Lotion

1 egg white (small egg)
50 ml (10 teaspoons) warm water

This completely unsophisticated lotion is a very old-fashioned recipe. To use, mix the two ingredients together and comb the mixture through your hair before setting it. This recipe could perhaps be improved with the addition of a few drops of essential oil or eau-de-Cologne to add a little sweet fragrance to the mix.

Sugar Setting Lotion and Lacquer

1 tablespoon sugar
100 ml (7 tablespoons) boiling water

Stir the ingredients together well and allow to cool. Spray this onto dry hair as a lacquer or use as a lotion.

HAIR COLOUR

Finally, your newly luxuriant hair may not have quite the depth or shade of colour that you would like. Most modern hair dyes are alkaline and are not likely to improve your hair in any way. However, a more gentle and completely natural approach can save the shine in your hair and a fair amount of money in your pocket as well!

Privet or Box Rinses
— for brown hair —

A chestnut tone is very attractive in medium-brown hair. The method used by the beautiful Venetian women, painted by Titian, was to make a strong infusion of privet leaves. This lotion was used on the hair as a final washing rinse. The ladies would then recline in the hot Italian sun waiting for their hair to dry, and presumably for Titian to paint them!

Another lotion that gives a shiny chestnut glow is a strong infusion of box (*Buxus*). Cover a handful of woody box sprigs and leaves with water and simmer gently for about an hour. Allow to cool and use as a finishing rinse. The Methodist preacher John Wesley maintained that this infusion would also cure baldness: I am promising nothing!

Darkening Rinses
— for grey hair —

Gypsies traditionally used strong tea as a hair colourant and tonic. The natural tannin content of tea temporarily darkens grey hair but leaves a natural looking colour. Medium-strength tea will add gloss and leftover tea works just as well as freshly brewed tea, so save the dregs! A sage infusion also adds shine to darker hair, as does vinegar.

Another option for dark hair is to use an infusion of elderberries. This adds a deep mahogany hue to dark hair – make up an infusion and use as an after-shampoo rinse, leaving it on your hair for up to 5 minutes then rinsing well.

Rhubarb Hair Glow
—— for fair hair ——

3 sticks rhubarb (with roots if possible)
300 ml (1¼ cups) white wine

This is a most effective tint for mousey-coloured hair. With continual use, this makes the dullest mouse hair a lovely golden colour.

Chop the rhubarb roughly, place in a pan and cover with the wine. Bring to the boil and simmer gently for 30 minutes. Strain off the liquid and allow to cool. Apply to the hair and leave for between 30 and 60 minutes depending upon the strength of colour that you want. Wash the hair as usual. Keep remaining liquid in the fridge and repeat at the next shampoo if required.

Herbal Lighteners
—— for fair hair ——

There are several possibilities for those with fair hair. The most well known is a strong infusion of chamomile flowers used as the final rinse after shampooing. An alternative is to dry and grind up the chamomile flower heads and mix with hot water and an equal quantity of powdered kaolin to make a thin cream. Apply to your hair and rinse off lightly after the desired amount of time. To lighten your natural hair colour, leave on for about a quarter of an hour or, to get a warmer blonde tint, leave the paste on for up to an hour.

Another rinse for fair hair can be made by infusing saffron strands. This has been used as a hair dye for thousands of years.

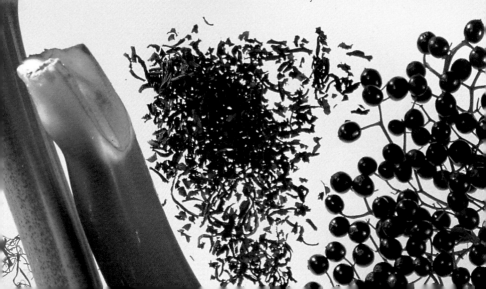

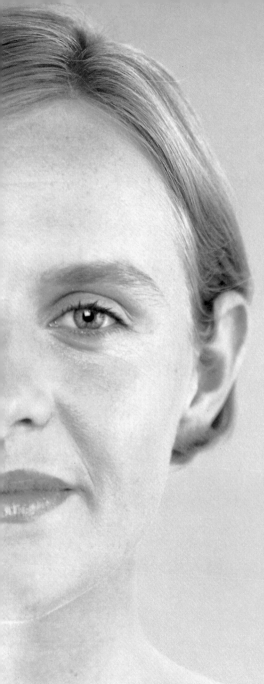

Face

A clear, glowing skin instantly shows how healthy you are. The look of your skin depends on not only what you put on your skin, but also what goes on inside your body and your general well-being.

What you eat will make an enormous difference to the colour and health of your skin (*see Part Two*). The body has to eliminate rubbish somehow and, if you fill your body with junk food, the skin is a useful place to eliminate excess toxins — hence the spots and blemishes.

It is important to analyse what type of skin you have, as this will alter the treatment it needs. A basic way to test your skin type is to blot your face with a clean tissue first thing in the morning (assuming you have not got a heavy night cream on). If the tissue comes away with oil on it, you have an oily skin. To test for dry skin, try washing your face with a baby soap and water: if your skin feels tight, you have dry skin. Anywhere in-between this, and you have normal skin.

Just to complicate matters, many of us have combination skin, with an oily centre panel, and the rest dry or normal. This requires a separate routine for both areas.

NORMAL SKIN

This is smooth, supple and often fairly young skin. It appears to have a satin, translucent quality and is everybody's dream. If this is you, then please take good care of a very valuable asset. Although you may be young, your skin needs careful treatment and a proper beauty routine — neglect will make it suffer very quickly.

OILY SKIN

There are both good and bad things about having oily skin. With all that natural oil abounding in your complexion, you may well stave off wrinkles for a lot longer than someone with very dry skin. However, oily skin does need a lot more cleansing. The sebaceous glands are working at double pace and so produce far too much oil. If left unchecked, this oil then clogs up the pores causing blackheads and spots, coarsening and enlarging the pores. Very regular and meticulous cleaning regimes are a must for anyone with oily skin or a panel of oily skin in a combination skin.

DRY SKIN

Dry skin is usually very fine in texture and often feels very taut. Flaking and dry lines are just waiting to turn into wrinkles if left untreated. It is important to feed the skin as often as necessary. It is also worth checking your diet, as sometimes this is a cause of lack of oil production and you can improve your skin from the inside.

A DAILY ROUTINE

It is essential to have a good cleansing routine so you automatically clean your face and neck before sleeping and again when you wake up. Taking care of your face will pay dividends in the long run. It is so easy to think you are too busy or that just one night will not matter, but it always takes boring spade work to grow beautiful roses!

The daily routine of cleansing must be thorough but relatively quick, as we are all rushing around and do not need a complicated regime that will take ages when there are only 5 minutes to spare. A good routine for any skin is to use cleanser, toner and moisturizer twice daily; and then once a week add a special treatment such as a face pack (see pages 50–55) or steaming (see pages 110–11).

CLEANSERS

Always cleanse very thoroughly at night when your skin will be dirtiest, and then again, but less thoroughly, the next morning. It is particularly important to cleanse twice in a day if you have oily skin or have problems with spots or blemishes. Choose a cleanser to suit your skin type, and keep trying different ones to keep getting best results. All these cleansers are simple to make and work just as well (I would say better) than many of the commercial brands available. Remember to always check a cream by applying it to a small area before using it until you are sure that it will not irritate your skin.

Honey Cleansing Milk
—— for normal skin ——

30 ml (2 tablespoons) warm milk
5 ml (1 teaspoon) runny honey

Blend the ingredients together with a small whisk or fork until it is a thin lotion. Then, using cotton wool or your fingertips, rub the lotion all over your face and neck. Rinse off with witch hazel, rose water or just plain water.

Lemon Cleanser
—— for normal skin ——

10 ml (2 teaspoons) olive oil
5 ml (1 teaspoon) almond oil
5 ml (1 teaspoon) lanolin
2.5 ml (½ teaspoon) fresh lemon juice

Mix all the ingredients together with a small whisk or fork until completely combined. Apply to your face and neck with cotton wool; then remove with tepid water.

Avocado Cream
—— for normal skin ——

10 g (1 teaspoon) beeswax granules
15 ml (1 tablespoon) lanolin
100 ml (7 tablespoons) avocado oil
60 ml (4 tablespoons) rose water

This can also be made up with almond oil – both work well.

Put the beeswax, avocado oil and lanolin into a bain-marie and stir with a small whisk or fork until the mixture is quite smooth. Warm the rose water to about the same temperature as the oil mixture. Remove the oil mixture from the water bath and add the rose water. Now whisk rapidly, preferably with an electric, hand-held mixer, until it has set. Pot and keep in the fridge or a cool dark place. Apply with a pad of cotton wool to gently cleanse the skin. Remove with tepid water.

Cucumber Cream
—— for normal skin ——

30 g (3 teaspoons) beeswax granules
20 ml (4 teaspoons) almond oil
25 ml (5 teaspoons) baby (mineral) oil
¼ cucumber
5 ml (1 teaspoon) glycerine
pinch of borax

This is a lovely cool cleanser for the end of the day.

Place the beeswax and oils into a bain-marie. Heat slowly to melt and stir gently to combine these ingredients. Juice the cucumber in a fruit juice extractor or peel, liquidize and strain if you do not have a juicer.

In a separate bowl over the heat, mix the cucumber juice, glycerine and borax, making sure the borax dissolves completely. Once both bowls are dissolved and warm, slowly add the cucumber mixture to the oil mixture. Add this very slowly and stir constantly. When all the juice mixture is incorporated, take off the heat and beat well until the mixture is cool. This must be kept in the fridge because it contains fresh cucumber. Apply with cotton wool and remove thoroughly with tepid water.

Lavender and Almond Cleanser
—— for oily skin ——

60 g (2 tablespoons) beeswax granules
15 ml (1 tablespoon) almond oil
15 ml (1 tablespoon) mineral water
1 drop lavender essential oil

Melt the beeswax granules and almond oil together very gently. Take them off the heat and add the other two ingredients, whisking them all together rapidly. Once it has turned into a cream, put into a sterilized and dried pot. Gently apply to your face with cotton wool or a tissue. Remove with any gentle toner or with water.

Almond Cream Cleanser
—— for oily skin ——

2 tablespoons ground almonds
150 ml (⅔ cup) mineral water

Put the almonds and water into a blender or food processor and blend for a couple of minutes. Strain through muslin or cheesecloth, and bottle. Apply to the face with cotton wool and leave for a few minutes before removing with water or rose water.

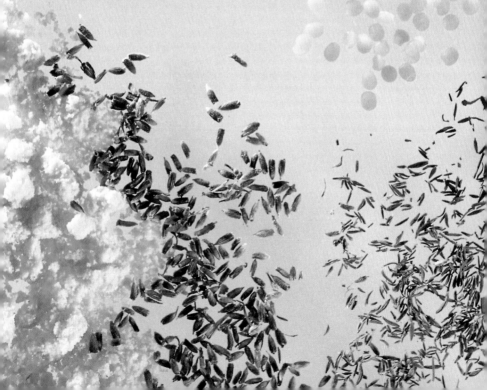

Mint and Thyme Cleanser
—— for oily skin ——

15 ml (1 tablespoon) thyme infusion
15 ml (1 tablespoon) mint infusion
15 ml (1 tablespoon) milk
1 heaped teaspoon wholemeal flour
1 level teaspoon cornflour or cornstarch

For the infusions, use 30 g (1 oz) of dried herb to 600 ml (2½ cups) of boiling water and leave to steep for at least an hour. Keep any unused infusion in the fridge.

Put all the ingredients except the infusions into a steep-sided bowl or wide-necked glass jar standing in boiling water. Stir until it begins to thicken. Add 1 tablespoon of each infusion and allow to cool. Pot and keep in the fridge.

Massage gently into your face with cotton wool and remove with toner or rose water.

Watercress Complexion Milk
—— for oily skin ——

1 large handful watercress stems and
leaves
300 ml (1¼ cups) water or milk
5 ml (1 teaspoon) honey

This will remove even more of the impurities and soften the skin beautifully.

Scrunch the watercress in your hands to bruise it, and add to a pan with the water or milk. Simmer for about 10 minutes, then add the honey. Stir well and, when the honey has dissolved, strain the liquid. Once the liquid has cooled, pour into a bottle.

Use by removing make-up with a stronger cleanser and then applying this to your face and neck. Leave the lotion on until it is completely dry then rinse off with water or a gentle toner.

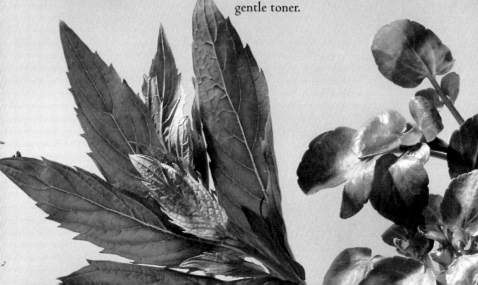

Lavender Cleansing Lotion
—— for dry skin ——

7.5 ml (½ tablespoon) lanolin
15 ml (1 tablespoon) petroleum jelly
(Vaseline)
60 ml (4 tablespoons) baby (mineral) oil
150 ml (⅔ cup) hot water
5 drops lavender essential oil

This cleanser is quite heavy, but softens the skin well.

Put all the ingredients into a bain-marie and whisk with a small beater or fork. Apply lavishly to your face and neck, then gently wipe off with cotton wool. Follow with a very mild toner.

Olive Oil Cleanser
—— for dry skin ——

10 ml (2 teaspoons) olive oil
5 ml (1 teaspoon) runny honey

This recipe could not be easier, and the cleanser works brilliantly.

Simply mix the two ingredients together until well combined. Then apply to the face and neck rubbing in well with the pads of your fingers. Rinse off with a mild herbal infusion or tepid water.

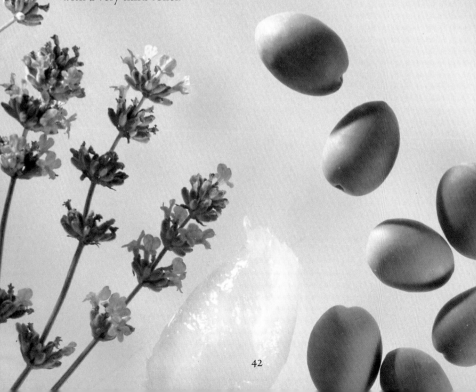

Traditional Cold Cream
for dry skin

40 g (4 teaspoons) beeswax granules
30 ml (2 tablespoons) lanolin
60 ml (4 tablespoons) almond or
sunflower oil
30 ml (2 tablespoons) baby (mineral) oil
pinch of borax
30 ml (2 tablespoons) rose water
3 drops rose essential oil

Place the beeswax, lanolin, vegetable oil and mineral oil in a bain-marie and mix well as they melt. In a separate bowl, mix the borax and rose water. Remove the pan from the heat and gently add the rose water mixture to the oil mixture. Then add the essential oil. Whisk well, until the mixture has cooled and thickened. Store in a sterilized jar. Apply all over face and neck and remove with cotton wood soaked in rose water or tepid tap water.

Lime and Orange Cleanser
for dry skin

40 g (1½ oz) cocoa butter
75 ml (5 tablespoons) almond oil
5 drops lime essential oil
5 drops orange essential oil

Place the cocoa butter into a bain-marie and allow to melt; then remove from the heat and add the almond oil. Add the essential oils and stir well. Pour the cream into a dry, sterilized jar.

Apply with pads of cotton wool, gently massaging into the skin of your face and neck, then remove with water.

TONERS

Regular toning is important to firm up the skin once you have cleansed. The toning lotion you will need depends on your skin and the type of cleanser you have used. If you have used a light, morning cleansing lotion and have normal skin, then it may not be necessary to use a toner. But if you have removed heavy make-up with a greasy cleanser, then toner is essential to remove some of the greasy traces. Toning will help close the pores and stop wrinkling and sagging.

FRESHENERS

METHOD

Make an infusion of the herb (*see page 16*) and allow to steep for about an hour. Then strain the mixture through muslin or cheesecloth and bottle.

Keep this in the fridge and apply cool with cotton wool to remove cleanser or just as a toner and freshener.

Elderflower Freshener
— for all skin types —

50 g (2 oz) fresh elderflowers (or 25 g/1 oz if dried)
600 ml (2½ cups) boiling water

This recipe works best with fresh elderflowers, so it is worth trying to get hold of some, if they are available.

Parsley Freshener
— for all skin types —

25 g (1 oz) parsley leaves
600 ml (2½ cups) boiling water

This parsley infusion is lovely and refreshing used from the fridge.

Lavender Freshener
— for normal to oily skin —

25 g (1 oz) lavender flowers
600 ml (2½ cups) boiling water

This is a particularly good toner for slightly oilier skins. It really helps if you have any spots or skin problems, and can help even out combination skin. The astringents opposite are also very effective for oily skin.

Lemon Astringent
──── for oily skin ────

5 ml (1 teaspoon) fresh lemon juice
30 ml (2 tablespoons) still mineral water

Mix together the fresh lemon juice with the mineral water. Pat all over the face with cotton wool either to remove cleanser or to tone and freshen skin.

Cucumber and Witch Hazel Astringent
──── for oily skin ────

¼ cucumber
45 ml (3 tablespoons) still mineral water
½ teaspoon borax
30 ml (2 tablespoons) witch hazel
150 ml (⅔ cup) elderflower infusion (see freshener opposite)

Juice the cucumber in a fruit juice extractor or peel, liquidize and strain if you do not have a juicer. Heat the mineral water and dissolve the borax in it. Separately, mix all the other ingredients together and then add the borax liquid. Mix well and pour into a bottle. Keep this in the fridge as the cucumber juice does not have a long shelf-life. Apply after cleansing, using liberally then blotting with a tissue.

Cucumber and Mint Astringent
──── for oily skin ────

½ cucumber
4 tablespoons fresh mint leaves
2 drops green food colouring (optional)
100 ml (7 tablespoons) vodka

The alcohol in this recipe acts as a preservative, making the liquid last longer. Put the cucumber and mint leaves into a blender or food processor and blend together. Then strain through a piece of muslin or a very fine sieve. Add the food colouring (if you wish to use it) and the vodka. Keep in the fridge as it feels lovely to apply a chilled, minty astringent.

MOISTURIZERS AND NIGHT CREAMS

Having cleansed and refreshed your skin, it is important to use a little moisturizer to put back any natural oils that have been lost and to add a little more, particularly for drier or older skins. If you have an oily skin, it may only be necessary to use a light moisturizer; night creams may be too greasy for you. But if you have dry skin then use a heavier night cream as well as a daytime moisturizer. Combination skins will have to choose from the various recipes and use a different set of creams on each panel of their face.

ESSENTIAL OILS

The simplest way to soften and feed skin at night, and in the morning as well for drier skins, is to use a combination of essential oils and base oil directly onto the skin. Almond oil is an easy base to use but you can also use grapeseed oil, or even sunflower oil, if it is easier for you to get hold of.

METHOD

Mix together 50 ml (10 teaspoons) of base oil with 5–6 drops of any combination of the essential oils suggested, or just one oil on its own. The simple fragrance of just one oil is usually my favourite, but two together can also work well, for example: lemon and geranium used for normal skin, lime and orange for oily skin, or lavender and rose for dry skin.

Use the finished oil like a night cream and gently massage it into your face. If your skin feels greasy by the time you want to sleep, blot off any excess with a tissue.

RECOMMENDED OILS

For normal skin:
lemon, neroli and geranium
For oily skin:
lime, orange and jasmine
For dry skin:
lavender, rose and calendula

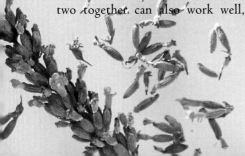

Creamy, Rich Geranium Night Cream
—— for all skin types ——

2 tablespoons cocoa butter
2 tablespoons lanolin
8 tablespoons sunflower oil
6 drops geranium essential oil

Place all the ingredients except the essential oil into a bain-marie. Mix gently while it all melts together and, once it has begun to cool, add the drops of essential oil and stir well. Put the cream in a jar and use as necessary.

This cream is also good for problem areas like knees and ankles, rough hands or anywhere that is feeling a bit dry and below par.

Essential Oil Moisturizing Cream
—— for all skin types ——

30 g (3 teaspoons) beeswax granules
25 ml (5 teaspoons) almond oil
60 ml (4 tablespoons) water
5–6 drops suitable essential oil

You can also choose from the oils suggested opposite to make up a personal moisturizer that is suitable for your skin.

Melt the beeswax in a bain-marie, keeping the heat very low. Once it has melted, remove it from the heat and stir in the almond oil. Heat the water, or use hot water from the kettle, and try to make it about the same temperature as the melted wax. Return the wax and oil mixture to the heat and gradually add the water, stirring constantly. Remove from the heat and, using either a fork or an electric beater, mix until it begins to cool and set. Then add the essential oils. Pot the cream and keep it in the fridge.

Rose and Honey Skin Cream
—— for normal to dry skin ——

7.5 ml (½ tablespoon) runny honey
3 tablespoons lanolin
1 teaspoon lecithin (available from health food shops)
60 ml (4 tablespoons) warm water
5 drops rose essential oil

Mix together the honey, lanolin and lecithin in a bain-marie. Once they have melted together, remove from the heat and stir in the warm water and drops of rose oil. Whisk everything together until the cream has cooled. Store in a glass jar. This is one of the few creams and potions in this book which is actually better kept at cool room temperature rather than in the fridge.

Lemon and Almond Moisturizer
—— for all skin types ——

45 ml (3 tablespoons) almond oil
2 tablespoons lanolin
15 ml (1 tablespoon) fresh lemon juice
5 drops lemon essential oil

This moisturizer has a lovely fresh perfume.

Melt the almond oil and lanolin in a bain-marie with the heat on low. Add the lemon juice. Take off the heat and keep beating until the cream cools and begins to firm up. Finally, add in the essential oil. Store in a sterilized glass jar in the fridge and use chilled.

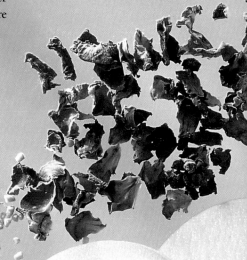

Devon Cider Apple Cream
———— for dry skin ————

500 g (1 lb) white vegetable fat
500 g (1 lb) apples (weight after being
peeled and cored)
120 ml (½ cup) rose water
few drops alcoholic tincture of benzoin
(preservative)

This is a less sophisticated cream that nevertheless works excellently. It also makes a good hand cream.

Melt the vegetable fat in a pan over a low heat. Put the apples in a food processor or blender and purée totally. Add the juice and pulp to the melted fat and stir together well. Remove from the heat and add the rose water and benzoin. Strain immediately, put into screw-top jars and keep in the fridge. Massage the cream into the face and neck.

Peach, Orange and Sunflower Moisturizer
———— for all skin types ————

10 g (1 teaspoon) beeswax granules
75 ml (5 tablespoons) sunflower oil
15 ml (1 tablespoon) glycerine
90 ml (6 tablespoons) peach juice (fresh)
½ teaspoon borax
5 drops orange essential oil

This can also be used as a body cream after a bath.

The peach juice can be made using a juice extractor or by purée-ing the fruit and pressing it through a sieve. Melt the beeswax and sunflower oil in a bain-marie over a low heat. Heat the peach juice separately and add the borax, stirring until it has dissolved. Add the glycerine to the oil mixture. Remove the oil mix from the heat and slowly add the peach juice, whisking with a hand or electric beater until the cream has cooled. Add the essential oil. All cosmetics with fresh fruit juice in have a very short shelf-life, so use it lavishly and always store in the fridge.

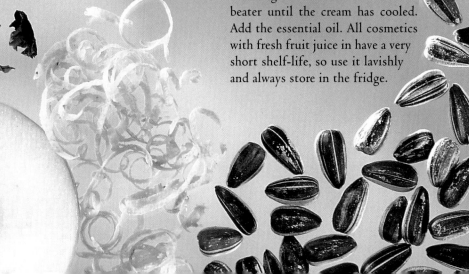

FACE MASKS

There are hundreds of different recipes around for face masks, clay packs and other lotions and potions to put on your face to deep cleanse and tighten the skin. None of these treatments should be used too often; they are intended to be applied perhaps once a week or, if you have a very oily skin, twice a week. However, when used correctly, they make your skin feel fantastic, clean, silky and smooth.

The quickest and easiest suggestions are those which come out of the kitchen. If you are having problems with spots and skin blemishes it is worth trying plain bio yoghurt on your face as a regular face pack a couple of times a week. There are also many fruits and vegetables that make brilliant face masks. Some suggestions are given below.

Strawberry Face Pack
─── for all skin types ───

125 g (4 oz) fresh strawberries
2 tablespoons powdered milk
15 ml (1 tablespoon) fresh lemon juice

This is suitable for all skin types unless you have an allergy to strawberries, so it is particularly important to patch test first.

Mix all the ingredients together into a smooth purée. Pat the strawberry mix all over your face and neck, and lie down for about 20 minutes; this can be left for longer if you have time – up to an hour. Rinse off with warm water.

Peppermint Pack
─── for all skin types ───

125 g (4 oz) brewers yeast
15 ml (1 tablespoon) witch hazel
4 drops peppermint essential oil

This is good for most skin types and helps to revive flagging spirits, making you more alert.

Mix all the ingredients together well and apply to face. Leave on for 20–30 minutes, then wash off using lukewarm water followed by a gentle toner.

Avocado and Lemon Face Pack
—— for normal to dry skin ——

1 ripe avocado
5 ml (1 teaspoon) fresh lemon juice

Avocado is a wonderful fruit, whose natural oils are great for normal to dry skins.

Remove the flesh from the avocado and mash really well with the lemon juice. When it is creamy smooth pat the mixture onto your face and neck and lie down quietly for 15–20 minutes, then wash off.

Vegetable Face Mask
—— for all skin types ——

1 large carrot
1 medium potato

This is a good softener that is made from easily available ingredients.

Peel and chop these vegetables and boil until soft. Blend them together to make a fine mash. Allow the vegetables to cool a little before applying to your face. Lie still for 10–15 minutes and then wash well with warm water.

Peach Cocktail Mask
—— for all skin types ——

½ peach (fresh or tinned)
1 tablespoon brandy

This is a really quick and easy recipe, but it is tempting to eat it rather than put it on your face!

Blend the ingredients in a food processor and then apply to your face and neck. Relax for 10 minutes before rinsing off with tepid water.

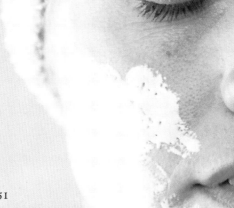

Orange Mask
—— for normal to oily skin ——

½ large orange (unpeeled)
30 ml (2 tablespoons) runny honey
10 ml (2 teaspoons) ground almonds
30 ml (2 tablespoons) double cream

Put the orange in a food processor and liquidize into a fine pulp. Add the honey and almonds and process just enough to blend the ingredients. Whip the cream and then fold the orange mixture into the cream. Apply to a clean face and lie down for about 15 minutes. Rinse your face well with tepid water.

Pear Pack
—— for oily skin ——

1 very ripe pear
1 tablespoon powdered milk

This is good for cleaning oily, spotty or generally irritated skin.

Peel, core and purée the pear, and then sieve the purée to get the juice. Alternatively, make pear juice with a juicer, if you have one. Mix the juice with the powdered milk to make a paste. Apply all over your face and leave for 20 minutes before washing off with tepid water.

Tomato Pick-me-up
—— for oily skin ——

2 tomatoes
1–2 teaspoons fine oatmeal

Tomatoes are excellent for combating blackheads and oily skin.

Purée the tomatoes and then sieve to get the juice. Alternatively, use a juicer, if you have one. Mix the juice with some of the oatmeal to make into a loose paste. Apply to your face and rest with it on for 20 minutes before washing off.

Parsley Pack
—— for oily skin ——

6 tablespoons chopped parsley leaves
45 ml (3 tablespoons) plain bio yoghurt
10 ml (2 teaspoons) cider vinegar

Parsley is good for oily skin, and also helps with spots and acne.

Mix the ingredients together in a blender or food processor. Place the green mixture all over your face and lie down in a quiet room where no one can see you for 20 minutes! Then wash off.

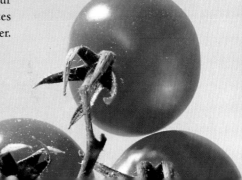

Pineapple Pack
——— for problem skin ———

1 fresh pineapple

Pineapples contain enzymes that help to heal skin problems and generally soften the skin. This is an ideal treatment if you spot cheap pineapples.

Peel and core the pineapple and purée the flesh in a food processor or blender. Once you have a pulp, apply to your face or any other part of the body you want to soften. Leave for 15–20 minutes, then rinse off with tepid water and use a gentle toner.

Rosemary Astringent Mask
——— for oily skin ———

15–30 ml (1–2 tablespoons) rosemary infusion (see below)
45 ml (3 tablespoons) kaolin powder
10 ml (2 teaspoons) glycerine
1 drop rosemary essential oil

This is a good face pack for deep cleaning the skin and removing old skin cells, leaving smooth, healthy-looking skin.

Make up the rosemary infusion with 4–5 tablespoons boiling water over 2 tablespoons fresh rosemary leaves. Steep for at least an hour then use as directed.

Mix all the ingredients together until it makes a workable soft paste. Apply all over your face and neck and rest for 15–20 minutes. Rinse off well with tepid water.

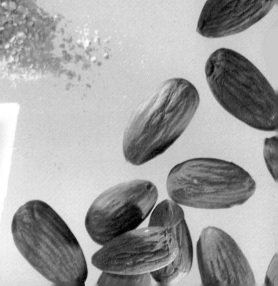

Carrot and Honey Face Pack
—— for dry skin ——

1 large carrot
60 ml (4 tablespoons) plain bio yoghurt
15 ml (1 tablespoon) runny honey
1 tablespoon fine oatmeal

Carrots are very good for dry skin and this should help to minimize wrinkles.

Peel the carrot and then grate finely. Mix the grated carrot with the yoghurt and some water to make a sloppy purée. Put the mixture into a small pan and very gently simmer it for about 20 minutes. If it dries out too much, add a little more water. It should now be the consistency of thick tomato ketchup, but a little lumpier. Stir in the honey and a little oatmeal to make a workable paste.

Apply all over the face and leave for 20 minutes, before rinsing off with tepid water and then using a gentle toner.

Leftover Rice Mask
—— for all skin types ——

2 tablespoons cooked rice
15 ml (1 tablespoon) sunflower oil
1 egg yolk
5 ml (1 teaspoon) runny honey
4 ml (1 scant teaspoon) lemon juice

This mask feeds the skin and leaves it soft and satiny.

Mix all the ingredients together and apply to your face – this looks pretty fearsome! Leave on for 15 minutes while you rest. Wash off well with warm water and use a gentle toner.

Apricot Face Mask
—— for sensitive skin ——

4 dried apricots
45 ml (3 tablespoons) plain bio yoghurt

This is a good mask for normal but sensitive skin and for any skin suffering from excess sun.

Liquidize or process the two ingredients together until they make a fine purée. If necessary, add a little water to thin down the consistency if it is not runny enough to apply. Rub into your face and neck and wash off after 20 minutes.

Banana Mask
for dry skin

½ ripe banana
10 ml (2 teaspoons) double cream
5 ml (1 teaspoon) runny honey

This is an excellent mask for dry skin – the only drawback is the temptation to eat it rather than put it on your face!

Mash the banana thoroughly and stir in the cream and honey. Apply to your face and lie down for about 10 minutes before washing off.

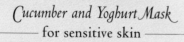

Cucumber and Yoghurt Mask
for sensitive skin

¼ cucumber
30 ml (2 tablespoons) yoghurt

This is a very mild pack, so is good for dry or sensitive skin.

Roughly chop the cucumber, put into a blender or food processor and purée. Mix with the yoghurt and apply to face and neck. Wash off after about 20 minutes.

Milk Mask
for all skin types

2 tablespoons powdered household starch
15 ml (1 tablespoon) warm milk
1 drop lavender essential oil

Mix these ingredients together until they form a paste and immediately apply all around the face, avoiding the more sensitive skin around the eyes. Leave on until it hardens and then wash off thoroughly with warm water, and use a gentle toner.

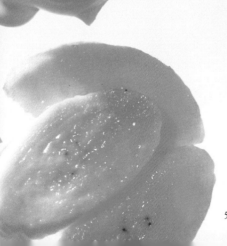

EYE CREAMS AND TREATMENTS

The skin around your eyes is very fragile. You should always be gentle with your eyelids; do not drag and pull at the skin when you are applying eye shadow. Likewise, the skin beneath your eyes should be handled with care; dragging it down does not help to get rid of bags under your eyes!

There are several very effective eye treatments that you can make at home and, as with every recipe in this book, by making them yourself, you know exactly what has gone into them. Many of the treatments also involve lying down while they get to work, which helps you to relax too.

It is important that you always use newly made infusions when bathing your eyes. Never use anything that is not fresh in case bacteria have developed.

Rose-hip Eye Bath
—— to combat bags ——

1 tablespoon crushed, dried rose-hips
90 ml (6 tablespoons) boiling water

Rose-hips make an excellent lotion to combat bags under your eyes. This is great before a night out.

Infuse the rose-hips for about an hour, then strain through a fine sieve. Soak two cotton lint pads in the liquid and then squeeze them out a little so that they do not drip and soak you! Lie down for about 20 minutes with the pads resting over your eyes.

Marigold Eye Bath
—— to soothe sore eyes ——

50 g (2 oz) fresh marigold flowers (or 25 g/1 oz if dried)
300 ml (1¼ cups) water

Marigolds have a wonderful reputation for soothing and healing. Use this to soothe sore, inflamed eyes.

Place the marigolds and water in a small pan and simmer gently for 20 minutes. Strain the mixture through a fine sieve, or through muslin or cheesecloth. Use this eye bath when it is slightly tepid, rather than when still hot. Soak cotton wool balls or pads in the liquid and gently bathe the eyes.

Rose Water Eye Gel
—— to smooth wrinkles ——

*2 tablespoons cornflour or cornstarch
rose water (as required)*

This moisturizing gel helps to reduce wrinkles.

Mix the cornflour and a small amount of rose water into a paste, then heat in a pan and add as much rose water as needed to make the paste a good workable consistency. Pot into a small container and allow to cool, then apply around eyelids and leave for about 15 minutes. Rinse off with tepid water.

ALTERNATIVE EYE PADS

Placing pads over your eyes is an excellent way to relax and prepare to look your best. There are all sorts of different liquids can be used to soak the pads, but here are some natural alternatives that come ready soaked!

Try medium slices of fresh cucumber placed over the eyes while you rest. Or another very successful natural eye treatment is to use slices of potato — use a potato peeler to get a thin slice. These will reduce puffiness and soothe tired eyes.

Alternatively, try tea bags. These make ideal eye pads. Soak them in warm water for a minute or two and they are ready to use. You do not have to stick to ordinary tea bags; there are many herbal tea bags that will work even better. Chamomile tea bags are excellent, as are mint, elderflower and rose-hip.

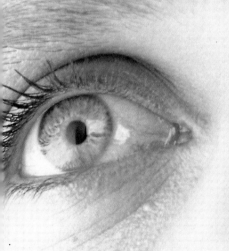

NECK TREATMENTS

It is impossible to forget your face as it stares back at you in the mirror. Your neck, on the other hand, is often ignored, covered up in the winter with high collars or scarves. Sadly, it is your neck that ages faster than many other parts of your body, eventually losing its tautness and sometimes gaining an extra chin! Keeping your neck regularly fed with good-quality, natural creams and doing a few stretching exercises on a regular basis may not work miracles, but it will certainly delay the signs of aging.

NECK CREAMS

The neck creams described below should be massaged into your neck every night, and any day cream or moisturizer you use should be brought down and massaged into your neck every morning.

Rose and Almond Moisture Cream

60 g (2 tablespoons) beeswax granules
90 ml (6 tablespoons) almond oil
45 ml (3 tablespoons) rose water
6 drops rose essential oil (5% dilute)

Melt the beeswax in a bain-marie, then add the almond oil and combine well. Add the rose water very slowly, stirring constantly. Remove from the heat and keep stirring until the cream cools slightly, then add the essential oil and stir in well. Pot and keep in the fridge.

Orange and Sesame Neck Nourishing Cream

90 g (3 tablespoons) beeswax granules
2 tablespoons cocoa butter
45 ml (3 tablespoons) sesame oil
30 ml (2 tablespoons) almond oil
6 drops orange essential oil

Melt all the ingredients together in a bain-marie, except the essential oil. When they have all completely melted and are well combined, remove from the heat and keep stirring until the cream has cooled slightly. Then add the essential oil and stir in well. Pour into a jar and keep in the fridge.

QUICK AND EASY NECK OILS

Either of these oils can be used to massage into the neck and moisturize the skin, helping the battle against wrinkles.

METHOD

Mix the ingredients well and massage a small amount into your neck at night. If you have put too much on and it still feels greasy after you have rubbed it in well, then blot off the excess with a tissue.

Citrus Neck Oil

5 ml (1 teaspoon) avocado oil
5 ml (1 teaspoon) grapeseed oil
6 drops geranium essential oil
3 drops lemon essential oil
3 drops orange essential oil
2 drops clary sage essential oil

Rose and Herb Neck Oil

10 ml (2 teaspoons) almond oil
6 drops rose essential oil (5% dilute)
4 drops lavender essential oil
1 drop rosemary essential oil
1 drop thyme essential oil

NECK EXERCISES

These neck exercises can be done sitting down on a chair with a back. Sit comfortably and, with your back straight, slowly roll your head in a clockwise direction, then repeat the exercise, rolling your head anti-clockwise. Do this exercise 5 or 6 times in each direction to relieve stress and tension.

Another exercise that helps this area of your body is to try to touch your nose with your tongue and, likewise, to touch the roof of your mouth with the base of your tongue — this brings the chin up and helps guard against sagging.

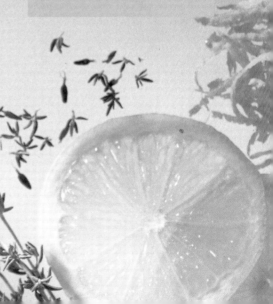

COSMETICS

Many of us are completely addicted to wearing make-up at all available opportunities, and the whole beauty industry makes an enormous profit every year because of this. Through extensive advertizing campaigns, cosmetics companies suggest that we cannot live without their products. However, many health and beauty books recommend that you forego make-up to give your skin a chance to breathe – well I have tried but, when you have been wearing it for years, it is not easy to cut back!

There are some simple ways in which you can help your skin, without having to give up your make-up. Try using lighter skin bases and less powder. If you can get your skin into peak condition, then you will not need heavy foundation, so it is worth trying to feed, soften and generally improve your face by using natural products.

Other areas of make-up, such as mascara and eye shadow, I cannot, hand on heart, suggest that you avoid. I would hate to have to lose my mascara and the scale of the cosmetics industry only shows that many millions of others feel as strongly as I do.

However, it is very important to make sure that you remove all make-up carefully and naturally each night. By doing so, you will give your skin and eyelashes a chance to recover during the night. One of the best cleansers I have found for removing mascara is almond oil; this can shift even the stubborn waterproof varieties.

There are few reference books on making your own coloured cosmetics, and those tend to use complex ingredients and chemicals which are off-putting to most people.

However, if you would like to persevere with some home chemistry, it would be well worth borrowing a book from your local library, or searching through some second-hand bookshops, as this seems to be a more fertile ground for such topics.

The only area for which suitable natural cosmetic ideas are abundant is for lip balms. The most basic lip gloss, of course, is just to put a little petroleum jelly over your lips or over a base coat of lipstick. However, if you want to be a little more adventurous, try some of the suggestions opposite.

Quick and Easy Lip Salve 1

petroleum jelly (Vaseline)
lanolin

This gives a very high gloss to a basic coat of everyday lipstick, and is good to use outside to protect your lips from the elements.

Mix together equal quantities of petroleum jelly and lanolin. Pot into a small container.

Quick and Easy Lip Salve 2

4 teaspoons lanolin
2 ml (40 drops) castor oil

When I made this recipe, I measured out the castor oil by drawing it up into a syringe, but you could use the small end of a child's medicine spoon which normally measures 2.5 ml, so use a scant measure.

Mix the two ingredients together and pot. Again, this is a very simple, but effective lip balm.

Rosemary Lip Salve

30 g (1 tablespoon) beeswax
15 ml (1 tablespoon) grapeseed oil
1 drop rosemary essential oil

Melt all the ingredients in a bain-marie. Pour into a small container and use for chapped lips.

Orange Lip Balm

30 g (1 tablespoon) beeswax granules
15 ml (1 tablespoon) sweet almond oil
2 drops orange essential oil

You could also use grapefruit or lemon essential oil in this recipe.

Put the beeswax into a bain-marie and melt it together with the almond oil. When the mixture has cooled a little, add the orange essential oil.

Honey and Rose Water Lip Cream

30 ml (2 tablespoons) runny honey
2.5 ml (½ teaspoon) rose water

Mix the two ingredients together thoroughly and pot into a small container. This is an excellent softener for lips – but is also very tempting to lick off!

Honey Lip Salve

10 g (1 teaspoon) beeswax granules
15 ml (1 tablespoon) honey
10 ml (2 teaspoons) almond oil

Melt the beeswax in a bain-marie. Then add the honey to the melted beeswax in a small screw-topped jar; and add the almond oil, shaking well until the ingredients are thoroughly mixed. This should be used every night, and is easiest applied using a lip brush.

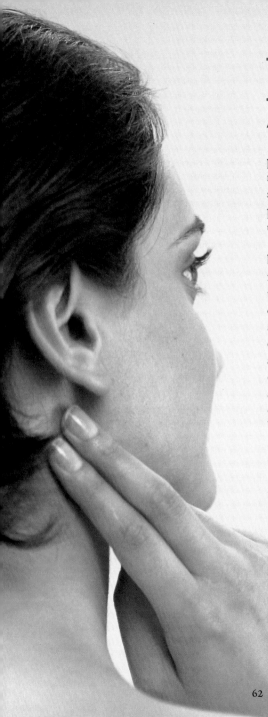

Perfume

The actual value of commercial perfume is as nothing in comparison to the cost of the brand imaging and advertizing. This should, therefore, make it an ideal product to make at home with natural ingredients.

There are, however, two drawbacks with making your own perfumes at home. Firstly, removing the oil from plants and flowers is a complicated process, so we will take some shortcuts by using essential oils, which still involves a certain amount of investment. The second drawback is that (assuming you are as brainwashed as myself by some of the glamorous adverts) nothing beats the feeling of treating yourself to a special bottle of perfume on a grey day!

So do not seek to replace commercial perfumes; just make some simple but lovely fragrances of your own that you can perhaps afford to be a little more lavish with! At least with homemade perfumes, you really can avoid any ingredients that include testing on animals or any other contentious issues.

HERBAL WATERS

Here are some suggestions for making your own herbal water, which can be used with great abandon after a bath or shower as it is very weak and acts as a gently fragranced body splash. It is also lovely used to spray pillowcases and sheets before ironing them as it leaves a lingering fragrance (lavender is my favourite for linen).

METHOD

Firstly, you will need to find a source of pure alcohol or a very high percentage proof vodka. 100 per cent proof would be excellent but is very hard to find, so aim for 80 per cent.

Place a large handful of fresh blossoms or leaves from the suggested list below into a large (approximately ½ litre or 1 pint) glass jar. Scrunch the flowers or leaves up in your hand first to make them give up their scent. Top up the jar with the vodka until it is just short of the top. Screw on the lid and stand on a sunny window sill and shake it every time you pass. Leave it for about 10 days and check to see how strong it is. If it is still too weak then try removing the old flowers and adding new ones for another 10 days.

Once you feel happy with the smell, remove the flowers and decant the liquid into a pretty bottle. Use this in baths to fragrance the water or straight onto your body as an astringent splash after a bath or shower.

SUGGESTED FLOWERS AND LEAVES

Lilac flowers
Lily of the valley flowers
Lavender flowers or leaves
Pinks (the stronger-scented varieties)
Lemon verbena leaves
Mint leaves
Rosemary leaves
You can also use many other varieties of scented herb leaves or spices such as coriander or cinnamon.

TOILET WATERS

Stronger perfumed waters can be made by using essential oils mixed with vodka, which saves on the time needed to extract the perfume from the plant. All these mixtures are blended to personal taste. You may want to try something much spicier or softer. Half the fun of making your own perfumes is experimenting!

If you discover a formula you like, do write it down, or you may never remember it. You can also make matching bath oil by substituting almond oil for the vodka and making a matching set of bottles for the bathroom! This oil can also be used as a simple perfume and dotted on the pulse points.

METHOD

Pour the vodka into a large, clean glass jar, and then add the various oils. Shake well and leave for 10 days to mellow, then check the fragrance and alter if you wish to. If you want a completely clear liquid with no oily residue, then filter it through a paper coffee filter.

Spice Island Cocktail

300 ml (1¼ cups) vodka
8 drops orange essential oil
4 drops jasmine essential oil
4 drops ylang-ylang essential oil
2 drops cinnamon essential oil
1 drop pimento berry essential oil

Exotic Vanilla Dream

300 ml (1¼ cups) vodka
6 drops vanilla essential oil
4 drops jasmine essential oil
4 drops ylang-ylang essential oil
3 drops cinnamon essential oil
3 drops ginger essential oil

Cottage Garden Bouquet

300 ml (1¼ cups) vodka
6 drops lavender essential oil
4 drops rose essential oil (5% dilute)
2 drops bergamot essential oil
1 drop mint essential oil
1 drop rosemary essential oil

Citrus Orchard

300 ml (1¼ cups) vodka
4 drops bergamot essential oil
4 drops lime essential oil
4 drops orange essential oil
2 drops lemon essential oil
2 drops rosemary essential oil
1 drop mint essential oil

CREAM PERFUMES

Cream perfumes make an interesting alternative to using toilet waters. For any of these recipes you could substitute your favourite perfume or your favourite essential oils instead of the fragrances suggested. In this way you can make a cream perfume to match other products you use.

METHOD

Melt the beeswax in a bain-marie and gradually add the almond oil to it until the two are fully blended. Beat together well with a small whisk as you slowly add the water. Remove from the heat and allow to cool slightly before adding in the essential oils.

Whisk in the essential oils until all the ingredients are well combined. Pour into small containers.

The Citrus Garden and Spiced Lavender fragrances have a strong, long-lasting scent and should be applied to the pulse points, while the Victorian Souvenir can be used more lavishly.

Citrus Garden

60 g (2 tablespoons) beeswax granules
30 ml (2 tablespoons) almond oil
30 ml (2 tablespoons) still mineral water
5 ml (1 teaspoon) sweet orange
essential oil
½ teaspoon lavender essential oil
½ teaspoon bergamot essential oil

Spiced Lavender

60 g (2 tablespoons) beeswax granules
30 ml (2 tablespoons) almond oil
30 ml (2 tablespoons) still mineral water
7.5 ml (½ tablespoon) lavender essential oil
2.5 ml (½ teaspoon) bergamot essential oil
6 drops clove essential oil

Gently Fragranced Victorian Souvenir

60 g (2 tablespoons) beeswax granules
30 ml (2 tablespoons) almond oil
30 ml (2 tablespoons) still mineral water
5 drops rose geranium essential oil
5 drops patchouli essential oil

The great thing about this gentle cream perfume is that you can use it very lavishly; it feels wonderful but will not overpower everyone when you walk into the room – a lovely fragrance just floats around you for a few hours! Again, substitute any essential oils you prefer.

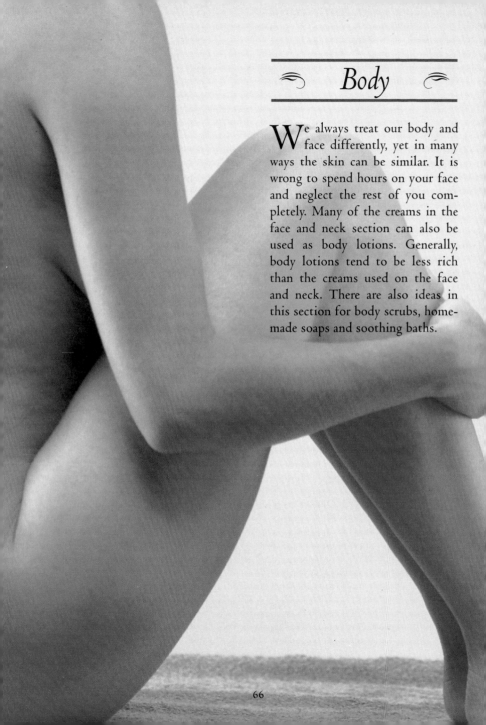

Body

We always treat our body and face differently, yet in many ways the skin can be similar. It is wrong to spend hours on your face and neglect the rest of you completely. Many of the creams in the face and neck section can also be used as body lotions. Generally, body lotions tend to be less rich than the creams used on the face and neck. There are also ideas in this section for body scrubs, homemade soaps and soothing baths.

BODY SCRUBS AND EXFOLIANTS

A very effective way to smooth the skin on many parts of your body is to use a body scrub. There are various natural products that you can use for this as you will see below. Bear in mind that all the face masks and packs in the face section could just as easily be used on your body if there is a patch you want to work on.

One way to wake up your skin and circulation is to give yourself a dry bath. Use a dry loofah and brush your skin vigorously to get rid of dead skin. Take care with the more sensitive areas of the body and concentrate on the tougher areas like back, legs and outer arms. Then apply a body oil or light lotion to most areas and rub off any excess before getting dressed. If you find this too harsh then scrub yourself well with the loofah whilst in the bath as this softens the actions.

Strawberry Body Mask
—— for arms and backs ——

250 g (8 oz) strawberries
30 ml (2 tablespoons) cream (any type)

Try this on your back, your upper arms, or whatever area you want to work on. Remember to patch test first, in case you have an allergy.

Purée the strawberries and stir in the cream. Do not try to treat too many areas at once as it will get too messy! Leave for about 20 minutes and then wash off.

Sunflower and Sea Salt Body Rub
—— for dull skin ——

small amount sunflower oil
sea salt

This is ideal for tired winter skin. It also works well if you substitute granulated sugar for the sea salt.

Treat your body in sections. First apply a little sunflower oil to soften and dampen the skin, then take a handful of sea salt and rub well into the area you have prepared. This will slough off any dead skin cells and leave your skin glowing and awake. Wash off the oil and salt mix with warm water: the easiest way is in the shower.

Lemon Bleaching Mask
— for dull skin —

2 tablespoons fuller's earth (available
from pharmacies)
5 ml (1 teaspoon) honey
23 ml (1½ tablespoons) fresh lemon juice
½ teaspoon ground cloves

If your body is looking a bit dingy
after a long winter of wearing thick
clothes, this bleaching mask will
help to brighten your neck or any
other part of the body – avoid sensitive areas, though.

Combine all the ingredients and
cover any areas you want to treat.
Leave for 20 minutes and wash off.

Coconut Body Rub
— for all skin types —

150 ml (⅔ cup) shredded coconut
150 ml (⅔ cup) ground almonds
150 ml (⅔ cup) oatmeal
45 ml (3 tablespoons) runny honey
rose water to mix

This is an excellent skin softener.

Mix the dry ingredients together
and add the honey. Add rose water
as required to make a smooth paste.
Apply to any part of the body you
want to treat and leave for 20 minutes. Remove using a flannel in firm
circular movements. Wash off with
warm water and moisturize.

Banana After-sun Body Mask
— for sunburn —

1 banana
15 ml (1 tablespoon) glycerine
5 tablespoons ground almonds

If your skin has had too much sun
then this banana mask is a good
way to put some moisture back.

Mix all the ingredients together
and add a little water if it is too
stiff. Apply to the affected areas
and leave for 15–20 minutes.
Gently remove and rub in a little
light body lotion.

Lemon Body Scrub
— for oily skin —

30 ml (2 tablespoons) sunflower oil
45 ml (3 tablespoons) fresh lemon juice
⅓ cup oatmeal
water to mix

This recipe includes oatmeal which
gives an abrasive touch to the paste
and is excellent for clearing the
skin. This is particularly good for
oily skin and spots.

Mix all the ingredients together
and add water as needed. Apply the
scrub to areas like the back and
upper arms, and leave for 15 minutes, then wash off with tepid water.

Kelp Body Scrub
———— for sensitive skin ————

3 tablespoons powdered kelp
75 ml (5 tablespoons) rose water
45 ml (3 tablespoons) almond oil
fine oatmeal to mix

Kelp can be bought in powdered form from health food shops, and is very soothing for sensitive skins.

Using a small pan, mix the kelp and rose water and heat gently. Add the almond oil and then the oatmeal until it forms a fine paste. Apply to whichever areas of the body you want to treat, using firm circular massaging movements, and rest for 20 minutes. Remove with a flannel, again using circular massaging movements.

Marigold Treatment
———— for backs ————

23 ml (1½ tablespoons) marigold infusion
(see below)
1 tablespoon kaolin powder
10 ml (2 teaspoons) glycerine

This is an excellent treatment for the top half of your back before you reveal it to the world in a swimming costume! Marigolds are good for healing the skin, and the circulation will be boosted by the massaging movement of removing the mask.

Make a marigold infusion with 25 g (1 oz) dried marigold petals and 300 ml (1¼ cups) boiling water and leave to steep for about an hour. Measure the required amount and mix with the other ingredients. If necessary, use a little more marigold infusion to get the consistency right. Apply to the back and leave for 20 minutes while you lie down – on your front! Remove with circular massaging movements, using a flannel. This may be easier if someone else does it for you.

MAKING YOUR OWN SOAPS

The best things about making your own soaps are that you can control the contents and choose what additives you would like to have, such as herbs and perfumes, and, of course, you can determine the size and shape of your bars of soap.

I never feel you save much money making your own soaps, as they tend to have extra luxury ingredients added, such as essential oils. However, if you had to buy a similar soap, it would not be cheap.

Making soap from scratch is a complex and often difficult process, using potentially harmful chemicals, such as caustic soda, which I prefer not to have in the house, as I have young children and animals.

All these recipes use a good-quality, pure, ready-made soap, such as castile soap. They are each enriched with luxury ingredients that no manufacturer would add: these creations cannot be bought.

Lavender Bath Soap

300 g (10 oz) plain soap
300 ml (1¼ cups) rose water
10 drops lavender essential oil
*3 drops lavender or pink food colouring
(optional)*

Grate the soap into a basin. Heat the rose water to boiling point and then pour over the grated soap. Stir well and, once it has all melted and combined, add the lavender oil and optional food colouring. This soap can then be rolled into balls to make individual soaps or rolled out between sheets of food wrap and then cut out with pastry cutters to give more unusual shapes.

Herbal Soaps

50 g (2 oz) plain soap
50 ml (10 teaspoons) herbal infusion

Place an infusion of your choice in a bain-marie. When the infusion is quite hot, slowly grate in the soap, stirring constantly as it melts – do not add too much at once. Find a suitably sized container to mould your bar of soap in and line it with plastic film or food wrap. Put the mixture into the mould, pressing it down to make a good shape. Leave somewhere warm to dry out for a week and then remove from the container by pulling the food wrap up. Then use, or wrap to store.

SHOWER SOAPS

METHOD

Grate the soap into a bain-marie and add the water. Heat the two together gently until they are fully melted and integrated. Then add the glycerine, remove from the heat and stir well. When the mixture has cooled slightly, add the essential oils. Bottle and use in the shower.

These recipes could be changed by adding any essential oil you like: such as a floral scent – jasmine, neroli or rose, or a herbal scent – lavender, sage or thyme.

Grapefruit and Orange Shower Soap

100 g (4 oz) plain soap
600 ml (2¼ cups) still mineral water
75 ml (5 tablespoons) glycerine
scant teaspoon grapefruit essential oil
scant teaspoon orange essential oil

Minty Shower Gel

100 g (4 oz) plain soap
600 ml (2¼ cups) still mineral water
75 ml (5 tablespoons) glycerine
6 drops peppermint essential oil

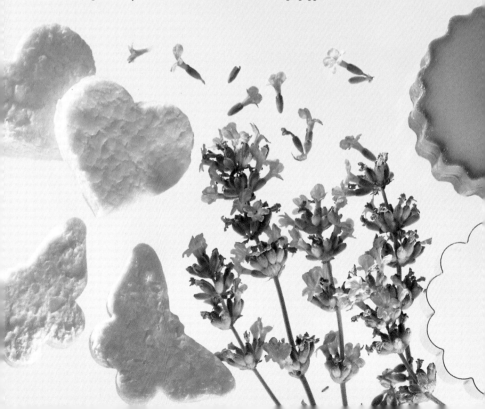

SOAKS AND BATHS

Although many people have given up having baths in favour of showers, there is a therapeutic nature to baths that cannot be found in quick and refreshing showers. They can, of course, be used for a quick wash, but far better if you use the bath as a beauty treatment in itself. Bathing was popular even before Cleopatra, and can still work brilliantly to restore energy and relax or revitalize you before sleeping or going out.

There are many real and apocryphal tales of famous ladies bathing in assorted substances: Cleopatra in her asses' milk for example, while others choose champagne and water from famous spas. All of these indicate one thing: that baths of any kind are good for the spirit. However, I think bathing in asses' milk is right out (unless you happen to have a pet ass), but milk baths can work just as well with a limited amount of milk and not necessarily from a donkey!

If you want to use the bath as a beauty treatment, then indulge yourself fully. If practical, lock the bathroom door so that you have complete peace and quiet, assuming there is someone else there to tackle any problems the other side of the door! Take a clock into the bathroom with you so that you can give yourself 20 minutes or half an hour of uninterrupted time without worrying about dozing off or forgetting what time it is. Try lighting candles and listening to soothing music to create a wonderful, relaxing atmosphere. Make sure you have all the ingredients you want, if you are planning a face mask or body scrub, then mix it beforehand and have plenty of cotton wool, towels and flannels for removing the treatment. Check any other lotions and potions you may want after the bath. Then enjoy yourself!

Lavender Bath

A simple recipe for a wonderful, aromatic and relaxing bath is to add 6–8 drops of lavender essential oil under the fast-running hot tap as you fill your bath.

Salt Bath

This could not be easier. Salt baths help to relieve tired and aching muscles and make your skin feel wonderful. Run a warm bath and pour 1–2 cups sea salt under the fast-running tap. Then enjoy!

Cleopatra's Milk Bath

1 ½ cups powdered milk (or 1 litre/2 pints fresh milk)

This will help relax and soften the skin. Lie back and pretend to be Cleopatra!

While the bath is running add the powdered milk under the fast-running tap. Fresh milk is also nice in a bath but the convenience of powdered milk is that you can keep it in the bathroom with a scoop or cup, ready for the moment when you feel the need of an Egyptian-style bath!

Floral Soda Bath

Baking soda can be used on its own to make a bath cooling and reviving, especially if you have been ill. However, it is much more enjoyable as a floral bath.

Fill a large glass jar (approximately 750 ml or 1½ pint) with bicarbonate of soda to just short of the top. Then add a teaspoon of jasmine, ylang-ylang or neroli essential oil. Shake the jar well and leave on the side for a week or two, shaking it every time you pass.

Use about ½–1 cup for a wonderful aromatic bath.

Cider Vinegar Bath

Try adding 1½ cups of vinegar to the bath – you can use cider vinegar or white wine vinegar. This helps to restore the natural acidity to the skin and relieves dry and itchy skin.

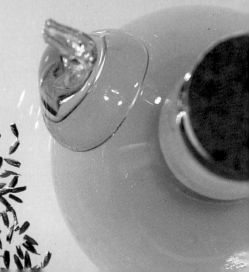

BATH OR TOILET VINEGARS

Although you can use plain cider or white wine vinegar in the bath, as suggested on the previous page, the herbal vinegar ideas below have an even more powerful effect. They are all very easy to make and, if you have a good selection of herbs and flowers in your garden, will cost you next to nothing. You may also like to try the short-cut method described opposite.

METHOD

Place about I cup of leaves or petals into a clean, screw-top jar. Heat I cup of cider or white wine vinegar to boiling point and pour over the herb. Screw on the lid and leave the infusion to steep for a couple of weeks, shaking the jar occasionally. At the end of the steeping time, strain the liquid through a sieve lined with coffee filter paper or a piece of muslin.

Use about ½ cup of the infusion for a wonderful, aromatic bath.

Rose Vinegar Bath

Use red rose petals for colour and any other varieties that have a strong scent. This makes a lovely scented bath.

Lavender Vinegar Bath

Use both the leaves and stems — there is as much oil in the stalks as in the leaves. This gives a pretty, old-fashioned scent that is very relaxing.

Lemon Balm Bath

The lemon balm plant is moderately easy to grow and, as a vinegar infusion, makes a wonderful, invigorating bath.

Scented Carnation Bath

Use the fresh petals of scented carnations or old-fashioned pinks, depending on which you prefer and what is available.

Mixed Herb Bath

Just choose a selection from any of the herbs you have growing in the garden that you enjoy smelling. The fresh herby smell of the bath is wonderful.

Floral Vinegar Bath

Choose any of the flowers you have in the garden that have a strong scent. Honeysuckle works well, as do jasmine flowers.

SHORT-CUT BATH VINEGARS

If you cannot bear to wait for weeks to try these herbal vinegars then you can cheat by using essential oils with vinegar. This can be done immediately before the bath . For every 600 ml (2½ cups) of vinegar you will need to use about 12 drops of essential oil. You can experiment with this if you would like your bath to be stronger or weaker, but be careful not to add too much essential oil, as they can be very strong. Rose, lavender and just a drop of clove makes a nice combination, and all the citrus fruits combine well with bergamot for a refreshing bath. Try exotic oils like patchouli and ylang-ylang for special treats.

BATH OILS

Scented oils in the bath add softness to your skin and a lovely perfume to the steam which works on your mind as well as your body. Do not try using baby oil in a bath as it is a mineral oil that does not disperse well and is not absorbed by the skin. Use any of the vegetable oils. Almond oil is more expensive than a basic sunflower oil, but you should try several different oils and decide which you prefer.

METHOD
Simply add a little essential oil to the base oil. The recipes below can be adapted, using any other oils of your choice.

Use 2 tablespoons of essential oil to every 5 tablespoons of base oil. Mix together and leave for a few days for the scent to develop. Use about 1 teaspoon in a bath.

Orange Grove Bath Oil
75 ml (5 tablespoons) base oil
15 ml (1 tablespoon) orange essential oil
7.5 ml (½ tablespoon) grapefruit essential oil
7.5 ml (½ tablespoon) lime essential oil

Jasmine and Ginger Bath Oil
75 ml (5 tablespoons) base oil
23 ml (1½ tablespoons) jasmine
essential oil
7.5 ml (½ tablespoon) ginger essential oil

Orange and Glycerine Bath Oil

50 ml (10 teaspoons) glycerine
240 ml (1 cup) water
5 ml (1 teaspoon) rose geranium essential oil
5 ml (1 teaspoon) orange essential oil
2.5 ml (½ teaspoon) patchouli essential oil

Mix together well and shake again immediately before using. Use 1 tablespoon in a bath.

Herbal Bath Oil

50 ml (10 teaspoons) glycerine
50 ml (10 teaspoons) almond or castor oil
5 ml (1 teaspoon) lavender essential oil
5 ml (1 teaspoon) mint essential oil
5 ml (1 teaspoon) rosemary essential oil

Mix together well and use about 1 tablespoon in a bath.

Old-fashioned Lavender Bath

2 tablespoons gum Arabic (available from pharmacies)
30 ml (2 tablespoons) sunflower oil
20 drops lavender essential oil
5 drops cinnamon essential oil
5 drops clove essential oil
240 ml (1 cup) water

Make a paste by adding the oils to the gum Arabic. When you have a smooth paste with no lumps, add the water a spoonful at a time until it all combines. An electric beater speeds things up.

BUBBLE BATHS

If you simply cannot bear the idea of a bath without bubbles, then the easiest and simplest way is to buy a good-quality, plain shampoo or organic dish-washing detergent. Then, simply add some essential oils of your choice to make it smell herby, spicy or whatever fragrance appeals to you. You may like to try the suggestions below.

Herbal Bubble Bath

300 ml (1¼ cups) organic liquid detergent
300 ml (1¼ cups) boiling water
25 g (1 oz) dried mint, rosemary and lavender mixed
5 ml (1 teaspoon) mint essential oil
2.5 ml (½ teaspoon) lavender essential oil
2.5 ml (½ teaspoon) rosemary essential oil

Steep the herbs in boiling water for about an hour. Then strain through a coffee filter paper or muslin and mix the resulting liquid with the other ingredients. Bottle and label.

Perfumed Bubbles

240 ml (1 cup) organic liquid detergent
5 drops bergamot essential oil
5 drops lavender essential oil

Mix together well and use about 2 tablespoons in a bath.

BATH BAGS

The final way of introducing scents and softeners into your bath is to use bath bags. These are little cheesecloth or cotton bags that allow you to soak fresh or dried herbs and spices in the bath to add aromas and soothing properties, but no leaves or sharp stalks!

METHOD

You can use any piece of thin cloth – a handkerchief might be the easiest thing to find immediately. Place a couple of tablespoons of your chosen ingredients in the centre, gather up the sides and corners and secure with an elastic band. Tie ribbon or string around the top of the bag and tie it onto the bath taps. You must have a long enough piece of ribbon or string so that the bag can dangle in the water as it pours into the bath.

There are many possibilities for the contents of your bath bags – try several from the list suggested below. If you are using dried ingredients then you could make up several at once and keep them in a pile in the bathroom, where they will be both decorative and ready for use!

Bran and Chamomile

2 tablespoons bran
1 tablespoon chamomile flowers

Almond and Lavender

2 tablespoons ground almonds
2 teaspoons lavender flowers

Rosemary and Bay

2 tablespoons rosemary leaves
3 torn bay leaves

Lemon Balm and Spearmint

2 tablespoons lemon balm
1 tablespoon mint

Pine and Mint

2 tablespoons pine needles
1 tablespoon mint leaves

Rose Geranium

1 tablespoon rose geranium leaves
1 tablespoon blackberry leaves

Rose and Peppermint

1 tablespoon rose petals
1 tablespoon mint leaves
1 tablespoon oatmeal

AFTER-BATH PAMPERING

Once you have reluctantly dragged yourself from your bath, or have hopped out as it became cold and unwelcoming, then is the time for body creams and lotions to finish the good work that you have already started with your bath.

Depending on your skin, you will need a different type of product to finish your beauty session. If you have very dry skin or areas where the skin is chapped or rough, then you need to use a heavier nourishing cream. If you have normal skin, then a body lotion is probably best. If you have very oily skin or just want to wake yourself up bit, then a body splash as a toner and astringent may be the answer.

Patchouli Massage Cream
—— for normal skin ——

4 tablespoons lanolin
60 ml (4 tablespoons) sunflower oil
2 tablespoons petroleum jelly (Vaseline)
135 ml (9 tablespoons) warm water
1 ml (20 drops) patchouli essential oil

Heat the lanolin, sunflower oil and petroleum jelly in a bain-marie. When it has all melted and combined, measure in the warm water and stir well. Take it off the heat and, when the mixture has cooled a little, add the essential oil, and pot.

Patchouli has a reputation as an aphrodisiac, depending, of course, on how much you like the perfume. However, having pampered yourself with this lovely cream – anything could happen!

Lime and Rose Water Lotion
—— for normal skin ——

45 ml (3 tablespoons) rose water
30 ml (2 tablespoons) lime juice
15 ml (1 tablespoon) glycerine

This is a new twist on a traditional lotion that my grandmother used (*see My Grandmother's Rose Hand Lotion on page 84*). The lime juice makes it less greasy and adds a delightful scent.

Mix all the ingredients together and store in a glass bottle. Keep this in the fridge as the lime juice does go off fairly quickly. However, if you use it liberally after a bath, this quantity will not last long anyway!

Try substituting lemon juice or grapefruit juice for the lime, or you could even use mango juice.

Coconut Body Cream
—— for normal skin ——

50 g (2 oz) cocoa butter
30 ml (2 tablespoons) almond oil
6 drops lime essential oil
6 drops ylang-ylang essential oil

This also makes a good outdoor face cream to protect against wind.

Melt the cocoa butter in a bain-marie, add all the other ingredients and stir. Package and use sparingly.

Rose Water Body Splash
—— for oily skin ——

45 ml (3 tablespoons) rose water
15 ml (1 tablespoon) witch hazel

Mix together and keep in the fridge. Splash onto your body after a bath to tone and refresh your skin.

Herb and Witch Hazel Body Splash
—— for oily skin ——

15 g (½ oz) rose petals
15 g (½ oz) lavender flowers
15 g (½ oz) rosemary leaves
15 g (½ oz) mint leaves
15 g (½ oz) lemon thyme leaves
75 ml (5 tablespoons) witch hazel

Warm the witch hazel and pour over the herbs in a glass jar. Screw down the lid and leave for two weeks, shaking occasionally as you pass. Strain through a coffee filter paper or muslin, and bottle. Keep in the fridge and use as desired after a bath or shower.

Vitamin E Nourishing Cream
—— for dry skin ——

50 ml (10 teaspoons) lanolin
30 ml (2 tablespoons) almond oil
16 drops vitamin E oil
12 drops lavender essential oil
6 drops clove essential oil
6 drops rose essential oil (5% dilute)

The vitamin E oil used here can be obtained from a pharmacy in capsules which can then be punctured to obtain the oil.

Melt the lanolin in a bain-marie and add all the other ingredients, mixing thoroughly. Package into a container and leave for a couple of days while the scents mellow. Use sparingly and rub in well. This is a lovely rich cream, so you do not need to use much.

Apricot Body Oil
—— for stretch marks ——

125 ml (½ cup) apricot kernel oil
5 drops cinnamon essential oil

This softens and feeds the skin with moisture; it is also effective in reducing stretch marks.

Place both ingredients in a screw-topped jar and shake well. Smooth on all over the body, but avoid using this oil on the face — cinnamon is a lovely fragrance but can be overpowering if used near the nose.

Traditional Rose Water Softener
—— for dry skin ——

125 ml (½ cup) rose water
125 ml (½ cup) glycerine

Mix the the rose water and glycerine together. If you would like a stronger rose scent, you can also add a couple of drops of rose essential oil. This cream is ideal for rough areas, like elbows and feet, after a bath.

Orange and Glycerine Softener
—— for chapped skin ——

125 ml (½ cup) glycerine
6 drops rosemary essential oil
6 drops orange essential oil
3 drops bergamot essential oil

This is a heavy cream that is not easily absorbed, but it does help to soften the skin effectively.

Mix all these ingredients together in a bottle. Rub well into the skin in affected areas.

Lemon Super Cream
—— for problem areas ——

2 tablespoons lanolin
15 ml (1 tablespoon) almond oil
15 ml (1 tablespoon) glycerine
2–4 drops lemon essential oil

Melt the lanolin in a bain-marie. Add all the other ingredients and then decant into a pot or jar.

DEODORANTS

Natural deodorants work by combating the micro-organisms or bacteria that cause body odour. They cannot, however, control perspiration to the same degree as the strong, chemical, commercial antiperspirants do. On the other hand, by using a natural deodorant, such as one of those described below, you can avoid many of the problems sometimes encountered with these stronger products, such as allergies, animal testing and harmful aerosols.

The best prevention for coping with body odour is frequent washing – at least twice a day.

However, some people have a greater tendency to sweat, whereas others can remain cool as a cucumber! One cause of body odour can be the food that we eat coming out as scent through our pores. This is why people who eat a lot of garlic or meat smell more strongly than those who do not.

The two natural recipes given below are both possibilities that have worked for many people over time. It is always worth trying out a natural product as it may be just right for you.

Herbal Mint Deodorant

1 cup fresh mint (eau-de-Cologne or spearmint varieties work well)
1 cup white wine or cider vinegar

Bruise the mint by crushing it in your hands and place in a glass jar. Heat the vinegar and pour over the mint. Leave this to steep for a week or so, shaking each time you pass. Then strain through coffee filter paper or muslin.

When you have washed in the morning, dab a little of this vinegar under each arm.

Lemon Deodorant

125 ml (½ cup) witch hazel
15 ml (1 tablespoon) tincture of arnica (available from a pharmacy)
5 ml (1 teaspoon) glycerine
3–4 drops lemon essential oil

Mix all the ingredients well. Bottle and store in the fridge.

Apply with cotton wool under both arms, twice daily after washing. You may find that you need to use natural deodorants more frequently through the day than the stronger chemical ones.

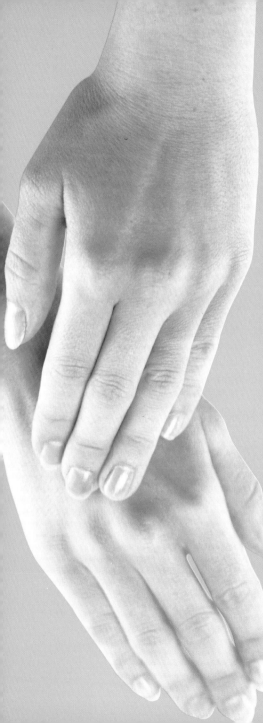

～ *Hands* ～

Your hands are always on show and, if you have spent time and effort perfecting your appearance, it is a big mistake to forget your hands. They really do respond to any attention given to them. You do not need to use expensive treatments as there are many excellent creams you can make at home – but do use them regularly.

Detergents and soaps dry your skin, and no matter what the advertizements suggest, frequent washing-up does damage your hands. Keep some hand cream by the sink to replace lost moisture and natural oils every time you wash up. In an ideal world we should all wear rubber gloves for any job that involves mistreating our hands.

The ultimate hand treatment is to use one of the heavy softeners opposite. Ladle it onto your hands before you go to sleep and then wear some protective cotton gloves all night. It used to be very popular to wear gloves at night – a habit I have not managed to cultivate! But, if you have very dry hands through too much dirty work like gardening or decorating, then this could be a good emergency treatment.

HAND SOFTENERS

The quickest and simplest way to soften your hands has to be rubbing 1 or 2 drops of glycerine into them. Although it does take quite a while for the glycerine to be absorbed, this is a very effective treatment, even if your hands are in a very bad state. It smells nice if you use equal quantities of lemon juice and glycerine, and is easier to rub in, but be careful using lemon if your hands are cut.

Another very quick and easy hand softener is made by mixing 1 tablespoon of white vegetable fat with 5 tablespoons of glycerine. It certainly works but may leave you feeling more basted than pampered! However, if you have seriously chapped hands, the treatment is more important than the glamour.

An alternative treatment for really sore hands is to soak them for 10 minutes in a bowl of warm water with about 50 g (2 oz) of salt added. Then gently pat them dry.

If your hands are really dirty, try washing the worst off using a good soap *(see pages 70–71)* and then mix equal quantities of any vegetable oil and sugar together, and rub your hands in this for 5 minutes. This should undo some of the damage you may have done that day! Then rinse off and pat dry with a soft towel or tissues.

Protein and Glycerine Hand Softener
for dry skin

1 egg yolk
50 ml (10 teaspoons) glycerine
10 drops essential oil of your choice

Whisk the egg yolk in a small bowl, then add the glycerine and mix together to a smooth liquid. Add the essential oil, combine well and pot. This will last for up to a week in the fridge.

Rose and Glycerine Hand Softener
for dry skin

30 ml (2 tablespoons) glycerine
2 tablespoons cornflour or cornstarch
240 ml (1 cup) rose water

Heat the glycerine and gradually add the cornflour to make a thick paste. Slowly mix in the rose water and keep stirring until it has thickened up a bit. Once the cream has cooled, it can be used straight away. Keep in an airtight container.

HAND CREAMS

You may find these hand creams more enjoyable than the heavier softeners. Try massaging them in using the Hand Massage described in Part Two (*see page 100*).

My Grandmother's Rose Hand Lotion
—— for all skin types ——

25 ml (5 teaspoons) glycerine
125 ml (½ cup) rose water

This takes a little time to sink in, but softens skin beautifully. Place both ingredients in a screw-topped jar and shake vigorously. Use every time you wash your hands.

Rose Hand Cream
—— for all skin types ——

60 g (2 tablespoons) beeswax granules
240 ml (1 cup) almond oil
15 ml (1 tablespoon) glycerine
175 ml (¾ cup) rose water
1 teaspoon borax

Put the beeswax and oil in a bain-marie and stir together until melted. Add the glycerine and stir again. Warm the rose water separately and stir in the borax until it is dissolved. Then add the rose water mixture to the beeswax mixture. Remove from the heat and whisk well until it has cooled. Store in an airtight container in the fridge.

Lemon and Almond Hand Cream
—— for all skin types ——

25 g (2½ teaspoons) beeswax granules
50 g (2 oz) cocoa butter
125 ml (½ cup) almond oil
90 ml (6 tablespoons) glycerine
4 drops lemon essential oil

Melt the beeswax, cocoa butter and almond oil in a bain-marie. When they are blended, stir in the glycerine. Add the essential oil, pour into an airtight jar and leave to cool.

Lavender Hand Treatment
—— for all skin types ——

5 g (½ teaspoon) beeswax granules
30 ml (2 tablespoons) almond oil
10 ml (2 teaspoons) still mineral water
4 drops lavender essential oil

Melt the beeswax and oil together in a bain-marie. Warm the mineral water separately and slowly add the water to the oil mixture. Beat well with a small whisk. When you have added about half the water, take the bowl off the heat and add the rest, beating very hard. Finally add the essential oil, and pot.

NAIL TREATMENTS

Your nails are made from the same substance as your hair – keratin. In the same way as hair, by the time you can see and treat the nail, it is dead. The new or growing nail is below the cuticle, and it can take up to nine months for a new nail to grow through. To keep your nails healthy, you need a diet that is rich in proteins and especially Vitamin B *(for more details on diet, see You are What You Eat in Part Two, pages 112–25).*

It is also worth giving your nails a manicure treatment once a week, mainly as a preventative measure *(see step-by-step Home Manicure, pages 106–7).* Well-groomed nails will prevent any problems like hang nails, in-growing nails and generally splitting and flaking nails.

Basically, a healthy diet and a little regular attention are the best answers for healthy nails. However, if you have poor nails, then by all means try everything to strengthen them. Regular massage of your nails with almond or avocado oil can help to strengthen them, and another solution I have heard is to take three kelp tablets daily. Beauty treatments are very individual and you may find one that works for you and, within a couple of months, your nails will be stronger. If it does not help, you have lost very little.

The health of your hair and nails is often a reflection of your health some weeks or months ago, so a good balanced diet and plenty of exercise is likely to have a generally good effect on all parts of your body including your nails.

Cuticle Cream 1

30 ml (2 tablespoons) petroleum jelly (Vaseline)
2.5 ml (½ teaspoon) glycerine
1 drop red food colouring (optional)

Beat all the ingredients together and pot. This works brilliantly and costs very little.

Cuticle Cream 2

2 teaspoons powdered lecithin
2 tablespoons lanolin

This recipe is very quick and easy. Simply add the powdered lecithin to the lanolin and combine the two together well. Store the cream in an airtight container.

Legs and Feet

Most of us feel that this part of our bodies could do with a little improvement. The best treatment we can give our legs is regular exercise, softening with natural creams and a happy life to help keep minor problems in perspective.

Feet, on the other hand, are too often neglected. They work so hard for us: walking, dancing, sports — all these activities take their toll on them. Yet, still we choose to wrap them up in nylon tights, thick socks and tight shoes. Only occasionally in the summer do we kick off all these coverings to walk barefoot.

Try to respect your feet. If something is wrong, then visit a chiropodist without delay. Give them a regular pedicure (*see Home Pedicure, pages 104–5*) and keep them soft with natural creams, and occasionally use a pumice stone in the bath.

DEPILATORY TREATMENTS

Many cultures do not agree with hair removal on legs or anywhere else on the body, but in many countries this is considered very normal. There are several ways to remove hair on your legs.

The quickest and simplest method has to be shaving. However, this does need doing every 3–4 days and also toughens the hairs.

At the other end of the spectrum is electrolysis, which is best done by a professional beauty therapist in a reputable clinic. This removes the hair semi-permanently, but takes time and money. Some people even go to the lengths of plucking out the hairs individually. This is not to be recommended, as (apart from the length of time it takes) sometimes the hairs twist as they grow back and become in-growing.

The middle ground is covered by depilatory creams and waxing. Waxing is a fairly simple operation, which pulls the hair out by the root and gradually diminishes regrowth. However, some people find this more painful than others. A natural alternative to waxing is sugaring.

SUGARING

EQUIPMENT NEEDED

500 g (1 lb) sugar
juice from 2 lemons
7.5 ml (1½ teaspoons) glycerine
strips of cotton or cheesecloth

This does take a little time and experience to get it right, but it is very inexpensive and leaves your legs smooth and satiny.

Melt the sugar with the lemon juice and simmer very slowly until it is a light golden colour. Add the glycerine and mix well. Use the mixture fairly warm, but not too hot or you will burn yourself. With a kitchen spatula, apply long panels of the sugar solution down the leg and press a strip of material into the solution. Wait a moment and then rip off the piece of material, pulling towards you and keeping it close to the skin. This should bring the cloth, sugar solution and any hairs away with one pull.

LEG CREAMS

Once you have removed the hair from your legs, in whatever manner you choose, then a massage with a natural cream or lotion will help the skin recover and seem soft and silky. You can use many of the creams in the body section, a hand cream or something from the face section. Here, however, are a few more recipes that are particularly good for the legs.

Carrot and Orange Moisturizer

10 g (1 teaspoon) beeswax granules
1 tablespoon lanolin
90 ml (6 tablespoons) almond oil
60 ml (4 tablespoons) carrot juice
45 ml (3 tablespoons) water
½ teaspoon borax
30 ml (2 tablespoons) glycerine
3 drops orange essential oil

Melt the beeswax, lanolin and almond oil in a bain-marie. In a separate pan heat the carrot juice with the water and add in the borax. Do not boil this mixture. Add the glycerine to the beeswax mixture and stir well. Remove the beeswax mixture from the heat and pour the carrot juice mixture into it. Whisk until the cream cools and then add the essential oil. Spoon into an airtight container and keep in the fridge.

Lavender Leg Gel

15 ml (1 tablespoon) glycerine
1 tablespoon powdered arrowroot
120 ml (½ cup) water
4 drops lavender essential oil

Melt the glycerine in a bain-marie and add the arrowroot. Pour in the water and stir well. Then remove from the heat and add the drops of lavender oil. Keep stirring until the mixture cools down and clears. Put into a small container and keep in the fridge.

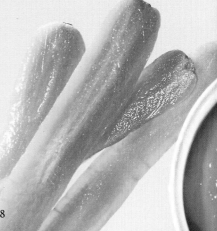

Rub for Aching Legs

125 ml (½ cup) almond oil
½ teaspoon white camphor essential oil

Mix ingredients together and use to massage legs. This will keep well in an airtight container. Camphor should be avoided if pregnant, or prone to epilepsy, asthma or high blood pressure. If in doubt, consult a qualified aromatherapist.

Rose Cream with Cocoa Butter

5 g (½ teaspoon) beeswax granules
45 ml (3 tablespoons) sunflower oil
30 ml (2 tablespoons) cocoa butter
15 ml (1 tablespoon) lanolin
30 ml (2 tablespoons) glycerine
100 ml (7 tablespoons) rose water
1 teaspoon borax

You may wish to adjust the quantity of rose water used in this recipe to make a consistency you are happy with.

Put the beeswax, oil, cocoa butter and lanolin in a bain-marie and stir until melted. Add the glycerine and stir again. Warm the rose water separately and add the borax to it, stirring until it is dissolved. Remove the beeswax mixture from the heat and add the rose water mixture to it a little at a time. Whisk well until it has cooled — an electric whisk is easier. Spoon into an airtight container and keep in a cool place.

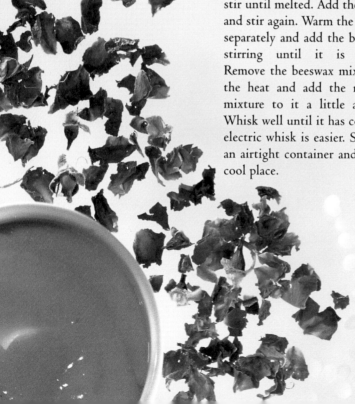

HERBAL FOOT TREATMENTS

It is important to give your feet regular attention. Try the Home Pedicure *(see pages 104–5)*, and the treatments described here. One way you can relax your feet is to use a herbal soak. You can even turn this into an instant massage. Simply fill a large bowl with one of the recipes. Cover at least half the bottom of the bowl with marbles and roll your feet around over them *(see also Foot Massage, page 101)*.

Lavender Foot Bath

2 cups lavender flowers and leaves
300 ml (1¼ cups) boiling water

Simmer the lavender and water together in a pan for 5–10 minutes. Allow to cool, then strain through a coffee filter paper or a piece of muslin or cheesecloth draped over a sieve. Add half the finished quantity to a bowl of warm water and soak your feet for 15 minutes.

Rosemary Foot Bath

1 cup rosemary leaves
1 cup salt
600 ml (2¼ cups) boiling water

Simmer the rosemary and water together in a pan for 5–10 minutes. Then strain through a fine sieve. Fill two bowls with water, one with cold water and one with hot water. Stir the salt into the basin of warm water and add the rosemary infusion to the cool water.

Soak your feet in the salt bath for 5 minutes, then soak them in the rosemary bath for 1 minute. Put your feet back into the salt bath for another 5 minutes and, finally, into the rosemary bath again for the last minute.

Briskly rub your feet dry with a towel and massage them with a little moisturizing lotion *(see Foot Massage, page 101)*. This should cheer up tired feet!

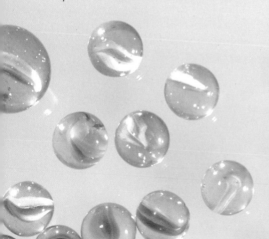

Rub for Aching Feet

45 ml (3 tablespoons) sesame oil
3 drops clove essential oil

This will help your feet to cope with tiredness and fatigue. Mix the ingredients together and massage into your feet well.

Patchouli Foot Softener

30 ml (2 tablespoons) lanolin
15 ml (1 tablespoon) almond oil
15 ml (1 tablespoon) glycerine
10 drops patchouli essential oil
5 drops geranium essential oil

Melt the lanolin in a bain-marie, then add the almond oil and glycerine. When they have all melted into each other, add the essential oils. Store in an airtight container.

FOOT EXERCISES

Exercising the feet should not be beyond even those who hate exercise. Sit on a straight-backed chair and circle your feet from the ankle, turning a full circle three or four times in each direction.

Also, try wiggling your toes, stretching them and spreading them all apart. This is another good exercise for the circulation.

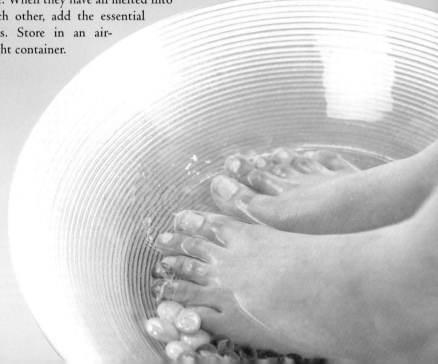

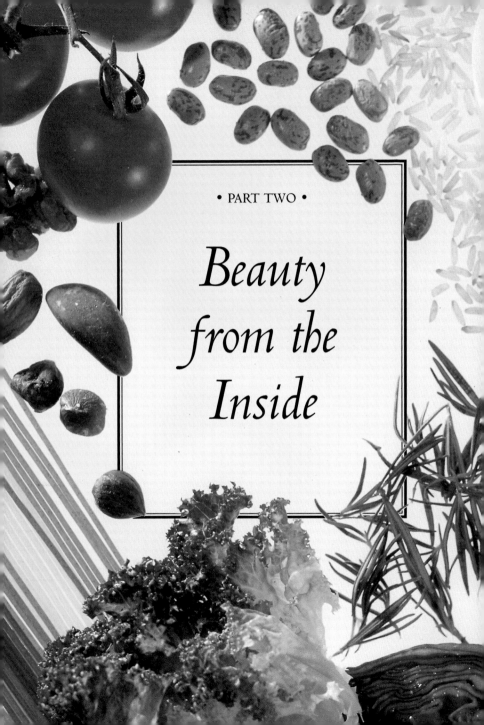

• PART TWO •

Beauty from the Inside

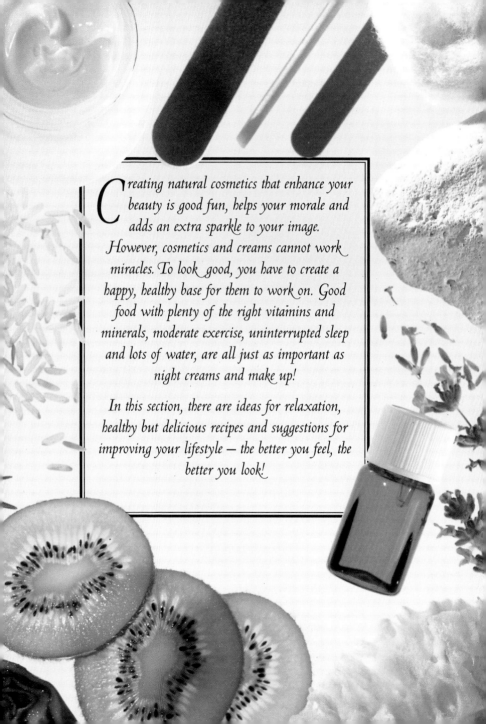

Creating natural cosmetics that enhance your beauty is good fun, helps your morale and adds an extra sparkle to your image. However, cosmetics and creams cannot work miracles. To look good, you have to create a happy, healthy base for them to work on. Good food with plenty of the right vitamins and minerals, moderate exercise, uninterrupted sleep and lots of water, are all just as important as night creams and make up!

In this section, there are ideas for relaxation, healthy but delicious recipes and suggestions for improving your lifestyle — the better you feel, the better you look!

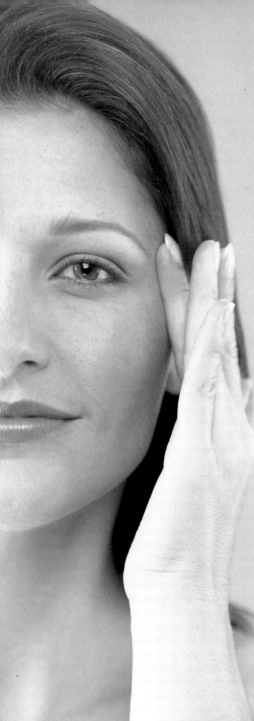

Time for Yourself

Never use the excuse that you do not have enough time to look after yourself. So many of us put other people's needs before our own and, in many cases, this is very noble. However, if you neglect yourself in the process, it will rebound on you as you become less healthy and probably less happy. Strive to get the mix right – it is the best investment you can make!

If you are constantly tired and under stress, it will begin to show in your face, general health and your body. A permanent frown line can develop across your brow. Lack of sleep through stress or tension can lead to bleary eyes and poor skin colour. If you do not take steps to relieve the accumulated pressures and to concentrate on yourself, then your body can fight back with unwelcome spots and rashes, not to mention fluctuating weight and a complete loss of energy and vitality.

It is only by 'trying and doing' that you will persuade yourself into new and healthier routines. Mental health, exercise and beauty care all matter and are each intertwined in the whole of your body's health.

RELIEVING STRESS AND RELAXING

Relaxing does not just mean sitting down watching television or listening to the radio. It means completely switching off, both mentally and physically. Try some of the techniques below – their benefits will show through your skin, your eyes and the condition of your hair. In fact, your whole body will respond positively.

COMBATING STRESS

Stress could be described as a continuous overdose of adrenalin. Adrenalin is very necessary: it gives your body an extra boost to help you run faster or work harder when necessary. So, although stress has taken on a negative meaning in today's language, a little stress is not a bad thing. What does the damage is constant stress – stress that builds up in an individual and continues day after day. Here are a few practical ways to help you cope with any stresses you may be under.

• Talk to your friends, talk to your family, and talk to your colleagues at work. Communication is very beneficial, and sometimes a problem that seemed insurmountable can be sorted out when shared. Friends and family are very important: nurture them and enjoy yourself with them.

• Learn to say no when you mean it. Saying yes when we really feel no, can often lead to a tremendous amount of resentment and stress.

• Make time in your schedule to look after yourself, and you may find more strength and enthusiasm for looking after others!

• Take Each Day as it Comes. There is no point in worrying about tomorrow. If something is worrying you, try to think of positive things you can do, and act on them.

EXERCISE

Exercise, generally, is very relaxing. Problems and worries can be forgotten while you run, walk or play sport. Exercise also strengthens your heart and improves circulation, feeding the extremities of the body, so you glow with health.

Any physical exercise that makes your heart beat faster for about 20 minutes will produce chemicals called endorphins, which actually improve your mood – so what are you waiting for?

RELAXATION TAPES

Another route to relaxation is to buy a pre-recorded relaxation tape. This gives you careful instructions for relaxation exercises that can be done at home. Find a recording by a reputable person and try to find a voice you can enjoy listening to.

You can also make your own tape by reading the relaxation exercise featured below and adding some calming music to make the tape about 20 minutes long.

SLEEP WELL

One of your body's major needs is the correct amount of sleep. Everyone seems to differ on the amount of sleep they need: from 4–5 hours a night to over 8 hours. You should know how much your body needs to regenerate and repair itself. Your eyes will never sparkle when they are deprived of sleep.

It is also essential to make sure that you make the most of your sleeping time. By taking some physical exercise each day you can make sure that your body, and not just your mind, is tired at bedtime. Also try not to take anything stimulating at bedtime like tea, coffee or alcohol. Instead, drink something soothing like a hot milky drink or a herb tea. Have a long soak in a herbal the bath just before bedtime.

RELAXATION EXERCISE

Lie on your bed or sit in a comfortable chair that supports your back and neck.

Calm your thoughts and try to iron out any negative feelings. Imagine yourself alone and content in a lovely place: a tropical beach, a country garden or whatever pleases you.

While you are thinking about the sounds of the sea, or imagining the clouds, relax your body. Start at the tips of your toes and clench each muscle and then relax. Work your way up your legs, then your arms, clenching and relaxing each muscle. Make your whole torso rigid for a few seconds, then relax. Finally, tense each part of your shoulders, neck and head, even your jaw and frown line, then relax.

Then play some calming music and be still for another 10 minutes, daydreaming about your chosen spot. Keep your body and mind completely relaxed, and your breathing deep and even. As you breathe out, expel all the tension from your mind.

This should help you to relax and unwind. Once you are in bed think clear, calming thoughts. If you are distracted by the problems of the day, try a relaxation exercise.

AROMATHERAPY

There are various ways that you can use essential oils to help you relax.

Some of the oils that work best in combating stress and promoting relaxation are listed in the Introduction (*see page 11*). You can use them in a bath; burn them over an oil burner to fragrance a room; have a massage with them; or make a steam bath to inhale them.

BASIC MEDITATION

Meditation is one way to find an inner peace and serenity. It also has good physical effects: your breathing becomes deeper and slower, blood pressure and pulse rates are reduced and, once you have made it a regular part of your daily routine, you will find an increase in your feeling of well-being.

If you enjoy the meditation exercises suggested here, it may be worth trying to find a group or teacher who can take you on to a further level. These are only simple beginners' exercises to give you a feel of basic meditation to see whether you find it helpful to combat stress.

MEDITATION EXERCISE

Sit in a comfortable chair – do not lie on a bed or you may fall asleep! Close your eyes and think of a colour – either just a blank square of that colour or, for example, a field of green plants. Try to think about nothing else and fill your mind with the colour. If you are new to this technique, it takes a bit of practice; you will find other ideas getting in the way. Just keep calm and return to the colour you are meant to be thinking about; eventually you will feel calm and peaceful. Try to keep this feeling and the colour in your mind for about 10 minutes.

An alternative is to use a similar technique to the relaxation exercise. Imagine a special place or journey. Close your eyes and remember a place you would like to visit again, and walk along that beach or country path. Look at everything you pass – the plants, flowers, waves or anything else you might be seeing – and really immerse yourself in the imagery. You will begin, with practice, to feel much more serene.

HEAD AND SHOULDER MASSAGE

Massage can be wonderfully relaxing, especially if you are massaged by someone else. Perhaps a partner or friend could follow simple massage instructions or you could visit a qualified massage therapist. However, try the simple self massage techniques outlined below: they should help relieve tension.

ESSENTIAL OIL MASSAGE

Essential oils should always be blended with a carrier oil, such as almond oil or sunflower oil, for an aromatherapy massage. The ratio of essential oil to carrier oil should be 6 drops of essential oil to 50 ml (10 teaspoons) of carrier oil.

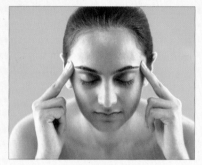

2. Rotate your middle fingers clockwise five or six times, as you breathe out. Good for relieving headaches.

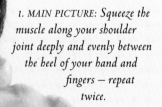

1. MAIN PICTURE: Squeeze the muscle along your shoulder joint deeply and evenly between the heel of your hand and fingers — repeat twice.

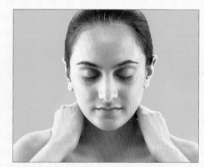

3. Relieve tension by rotating your fingers on both sides of your neck. Press firmly and work slowly down from behind the ears to the base of the neck.

SCALP MASSAGE

Massaging your head can help relieve tension in the scalp and also promote healthy-looking hair – your hair needs to be treated both from within and without to get the best results. Of course, someone applying the massage can be even more relaxing!

Many people swear by head stands and various other yoga positions. Try standing on your head for a few minutes and see whether you feel it has woken you up or not. I found it too much of a shock, but it may be different for you.

One way to massage your head is to stand with your feet slightly apart and breathe slowly but regularly. Lean forward from the waist, bending over until your head is just below your waist. Keep your legs straight and tap your head all over with your knuckles (gently but not too delicately). Then bring your head up slowly and repeat the process standing upright.

You may also like to try a 5–10 minute massage that gets the blood moving round your head and helps to boost hair growth and a general feeling of well-being. Use the heels of your hands and work over your head in smooth circular movements. Then slide your fingers through your hair from the roots to the ends *(see below left and right)*.

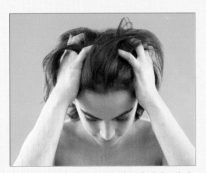

1. Place the heels of your hands behind the hair line, taking the weight of your head. Gently rotate them, and move over the rest of the scalp.

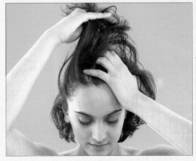

2. Cover the whole head, gently pulling your hands, one after the other, through the hair from roots to ends. Another good headache remedy.

HAND MASSAGE

Your hand contains many small bones, tendons and muscles, so take your time massaging cream in. This will help the circulation and alleviate tension and stiffness. Massage your hand with your thumb (*see below*). Then stretch your fingers as straight as possible and relax; repeat three times. Shake your hands; then relax. Finally, circle your hands from the wrist, three circles to the left and three to the right.

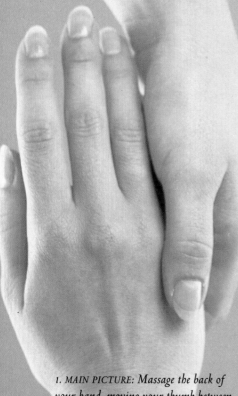

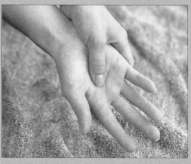

2. Make small circular movements on each joint, from the little finger to the thumb. Then massage the whole palm area.

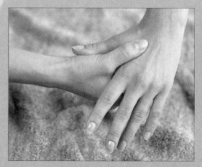

1. MAIN PICTURE: Massage the back of your hand, moving your thumb between the tendons. Start with your little finger and move across to your thumb.

3. Massage your hand from the knuckle, down to the wrist, again using small circular movements with your thumb.

FOOT MASSAGE

Foot massage is amazingly therapeutic – as any reflexology enthusiast will know. It is a bit complicated to massage your own feet with the same degree of relaxation, unless you have very long arms! However, the simple techniques described here should be easy for you to carry out on yourself at home. First of all, soak your feet in a bowl with herbal infusions or a scented foot bath added to the water.

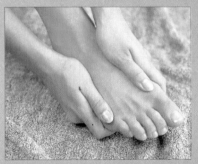

1. Placing your thumbs on the top of your foot and curling your fingers underneath, rub firmly along the length of the foot.

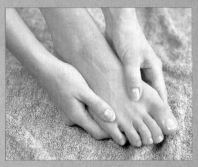

2. Then, using your thumbs, massage the end of your foot and down onto your toes, with firm circular movements.

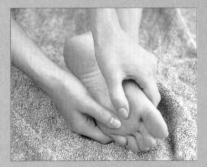

3. Work on the sole of your foot next. Rotate your thumbs with small circular movements, covering the entire foot.

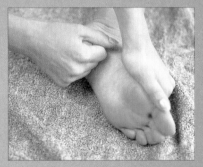

4. Finally, make a fist and gently pound the whole of the underneath of your foot, especially the heel.

AN EVENING FOR YOURSELF

A whole evening spent putting yourself first! I do realize there will be some of you thinking: *I should be so lucky!* But it may not be as hard as you think if a little forward planning is put into action. Most of us are happy to be in demand, but it does make it a special treat to have several uninterrupted hours to do whatever you like. If it is not possible then *compromise* – miss out the pedicure, skip the bath, whatever fits the time you have available. Life is for living and, if you cannot manage all of the plan below, do not forget the idea altogether. Just edit out the bits you are less keen on and enjoy yourself.

If you have family commitments that make it difficult, then maybe you could team up with a friend. If they could help you out on your relaxation evening, then you can return the favour on their night. You only need three hours and you will feel so much better, just by spending a little time on yourself.

EVENING MEAL

7.00 p.m. Start your evening with a meal that you really enjoy. This does not mean eating three family-sized containers of chocolate-chip ice cream and a packet of cookies to go with it! Plan a light meal so that you do not feel overfull, but have something you really fancy. Do not eat dessert yet, save it for later in the evening. Then allow about 20 minutes for the meal to go down before starting the beauty plan.

AROMATHERAPY BATH

8.00 p.m. Begin your relaxation evening with a wonderfully scented aromatherapy bath.

Have a quick wash before you get in the bath. If you are going to linger for some time, then it will be more enjoyable if you are fairly clean to begin with rather than wallowing in the day's dirt.

Run a bath that is fairly full but do not make it too hot. A steaming-hot bath turns your face red and is not very comfortable until it has cooled a little, so make it a medium temperature to begin with.

Once the bath is ready, add the essential oils of your choice. Add up to 10 drops and use either just one oil or a mixture of two or three, but no more or the smells become muddled and messy *(see pages 75–6 for some suggested blends)*.

Remember that personal taste is vital. You must enjoy this bath, not lie there thinking: This is meant to be good for me!

While the bath is running, pour a little olive oil onto your hair and rub it through gently. Then wrap a small towel around your head like a turban or wear a shower cap. This will condition your hair while you are soaking in the bath, making the most of the time you have.

When the bath is ready and you have oiled your hair, you may wish to add soft relaxing music, gentle candlelight and a cool drink in a pretty glass – preferably non-alcoholic. A drink does feel suitably decadent and increases the feeling that you are doing something just for you.

Do not stay in the bath too long; the idea is to unwind and soften your skin, not to turn you into a wrinkly, soaked prune! About 10–15 minutes should be fine, but again, this is your time so stay as long as you like: happiness is one of the strongest medicines there is. In the same way that stress can be very disabling, happiness or contentment can be extremely enabling.

TREATING YOUR HAIR

8.30 p.m. Once you are out of the bath, the next project is your hair. It will have benefited greatly from the oil while you relaxed in the bath. Now wash out the oil using one of the natural shampoo recipes *(see pages 24–5)*.

Once your hair is beautifully clean, use a quick finishing rinse on it by mixing a drop or two of essential oil with some water and pouring it over your hair. Rosemary is an excellent choice as it strengthens the hair and encourages new growth. *(For other finishing rinse ideas, see Hair Tonics, pages 28–9.)*

Comb your hair through with a wide-toothed comb. Dry and style it if you like; but, if possible, leave it to dry naturally, allowing it a break from artificial heat.

AFTER-BATH TREATMENTS

9.00 p.m. Having had a good soak in the bath, make the most of the fact that you will have softened all your skin, especially the harder skin on your hands and feet.

Start by massaging plenty of gentle body cream or lotion all over your body. If you want to use something really special and home-made, choose one of the creams from Part One *(see pages 78–80)*.

Once you have liberally applied cream or lotion to your body, then apply some more to the tougher places, like elbows and knees – they often need a helping hand! Next start work on your feet.

HOME PEDICURE

9.15 p.m. Poor old feet – all too often we take them for granted and, despite using them so heavily, tend to ignore them completely. Given even occasional encouragement, you will be amazed by how much better your feet can look and feel!

You have given them a good soak in the bath and so should have softened and prepared them well.

Remove any nail polish, and then fill a large bowl with warm water. If you want to add one of the herbal soaks (see page 90), they do feel good and smell wonderful. Alternatively, just add 3–4 drops of lavender oil into the foot bath. Place your feet in the water one at a time.

Gently rub your foot with a pumice stone, concentrating on the areas where the skin hardens, like the heels and the balls of your feet. Then replace the foot in the water and massage it well. Once both feet have been well scrubbed and soaked, dry them with a soft towel.

Rub a gentle cuticle cream (see page 85) into the cuticle areas and around the toes. Then press the cuticles down with an orange stick.

If necessary, trim your toenails with a good pair of manicure scissors or nail clippers.

Then apply more cream to the entire foot and massage it in well.

1. MAIN PICTURE: Using a pumice stone, rub away old, hard skin with a gentle circular movement.

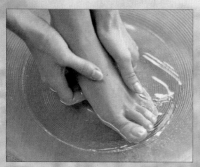

2. Place your foot in the water, massage away old skin and generally wake up your circulation!

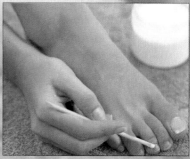

3. Having used a cuticle cream, push down softened cuticles and generally tidy them up with an orange stick.

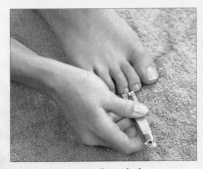

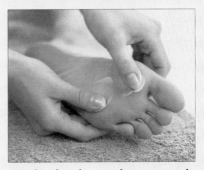

4. Trim your toenails with clippers; cut straight across the nail and then smooth the rough edges with an emery board.

5. Be lavish with a refreshing cream and massage it in slowly and firmly (see Foot Massage on page 101).

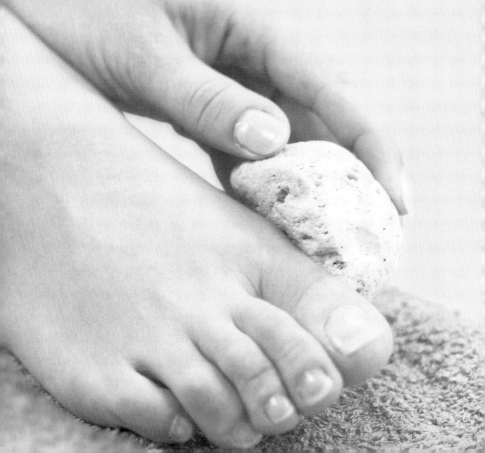

HOME MANICURE

9.30 p.m. Before you start your home manicure, remove any nail polish with remover soaked in cotton wool. If your nails are badly discoloured from constant wearing of coloured polish, try painting them with lemon juice to bleach them. Leave the lemon juice on for 10 minutes before rinsing off.

First of all, trim any of your nails that are too long with nail scissors or clippers. Then, using a good-quality emery board, file them into shape. Remember to file in one direction only as over enthusiastic sawing at nails will split and weaken them. Then rinse the nails.

Rubbing all that cream into your feet will also have softened your hands. Apply more cuticle cream and massage into each nail, especially round the base. Relax while the cream soaks in. Then, using an orange stick, very gently push each cuticle down (you can cover the end of the stick with cotton wool to make it softer). Be gentle as it is easy to damage a cuticle, which then takes several days to heal.

Soak your fingers in a bowl of warm water, then remove any cuticle cream left on with a tissue. Then apply hand cream and massage your hands for 10 minutes.

Now is not a good time to apply nail polish, as you still have the facial to do. However, you can buff your nails, which is much better for them anyway!

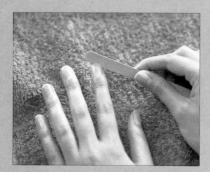

1. *Once you have trimmed your nails to a uniform length, file them gently into shape with an emery board.*

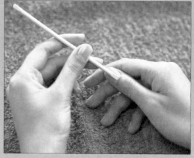

2. *Apply cuticle cream and use an orange stick to push each cuticle down. This should be done very gently and carefully.*

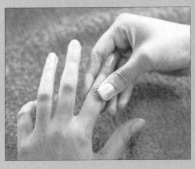

4. *MAIN PICTURE: Constant use of nail varnish can damage your nails and cause nasty discoloration. To get a really healthy, glossy look to your nails, polish them with a piece of soft cloth like chamois leather, or buy a commercial nail buffer. It is amazing how pretty well-manicured and naturally polished nails look, compared to varnished but slightly unkempt ones.*

3. After applying hand cream, massage each hand thoroughly, using the thumb and forefinger of the other hand.

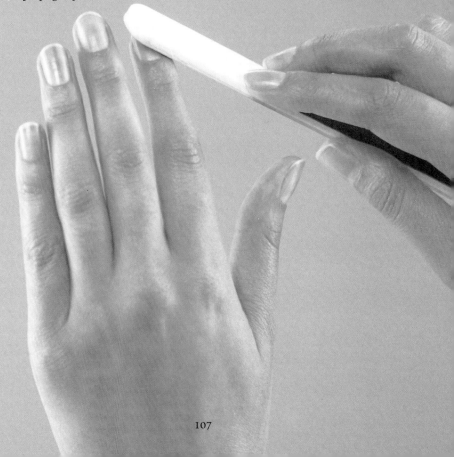

FACE AND MIND

9.45 p.m. Finally, having pampered the rest of your body all evening, we come to your face. Beauty often comes from inside as well as out, and it is important to concentrate on your sense of well-being as well as the skin! Allowing yourself some time for enjoyment will reap untold benefits on your looks.

First the outer layers. Cleanse your skin thoroughly. The steam from the bath and washing your hair should have opened the pores and started the cleansing process. Now choose a good cleanser, preferably one you have made yourself *(see pages 38–43)*. Gently and thoroughly cleanse your face and choose one of the face pack ideas suggested in Part One *(see pages 50–55)*.

Apply the face pack and then it is time to relax while it gets to work. Since laughter is such an important ingredient in maintaining one's health and happiness, now is the time to try it. I suggest that you listen to a tape of your favourite comedian or watch a video of a comedy programme that really makes you laugh! There are also many books that can make you laugh out loud. Alternatively, if none of these ideas appeal, ring a friend for a chat and a giggle.

Whatever your choice of entertainment, make yourself laugh or snigger for at least as long as the face pack is meant to stay on. Do not worry about cracking the face mask: none of the recipes in this book turn you into an Egyptian mummy, and a gentle face pack can take any amount of laughter.

This might also be a good time to have that dessert you saved earlier. Enjoy yourself for a while and, if you have chosen the right tape, video or book, you will go on smiling to yourself for some time after it has finished.

When you remove the face pack, close the pores with one of the toners or facial splashes recommended *(see pages 44–5)*. If you have nothing else, cold water can be used pretty effectively as a toner and freshener. Finally, apply some moisturizer or night cream to soften the skin *(see pages 46–9)*.

There is now just time to unwind before an early night. Have a warm drink – fruit or herbal teas work well, but have whatever you wish, avoiding strong coffee (this is not what you have been working for all evening). Now, sleep well – hopefully with a smile on your face.

A MORNING BEAUTY PROGRAMME

Although most of us would love to spend a weekend away at a health farm or beauty spa, it is not always convenient to find either the time or the money. You can, however, give yourself several mini holidays by taking time out for special mornings, evenings or even whole days, just for you.

It is always good to give yourself mini breaks, either a morning, an evening or, even better, a whole weekend. But never use the excuse that you do not have enough time to look after yourself.

Whether you are normally snowed under with responsibilities, or you are completely carefree, it is still enjoyable to take time to pamper yourself and start a whole new approach to your health and beauty.

For one weekend or weekday, whichever fits into your lifestyle better, decide that the whole morning will be for you; no chores no nothing, just time and attention for you. It is amazing how much better you will feel, and, with the renewed energy it brings, you will probably get as much done as if you had been working all morning!

As with all beauty plans or suggestions, you must use it with your own times and personal responsibilities in mind. Simply use this as a base to devise your own timings and programme.

WAKING UP

8.00 a.m. Before anything else, drink a glass of hot water with lemon juice (to taste) to wake up your system. Then try some stretching exercises. If you have an exercise video that you like using, then by all means use that or just play some invigorating music and gradually shake out and stretch each part of your body, dancing in time to the music.

Then get into the shower (or bath) and have a quick refreshing wash to wake you up and make you feel like facing the day.

BREAKFAST

9.30 a.m. Have a light but delicious breakfast. Fresh orange juice and cereal with sliced strawberries and bananas covered with fruit yoghurt and a sprinkling of flaked almonds is ideal and delicious. Alternatively, try one of the juices or breakfast ideas in the food section (*see pages 118–20*). Take your time and read the paper, or just enjoy the rest.

HERBAL STEAM TREATMENT

10.30 a.m.   Steam treatments are amazingly invigorating and deep-cleansing. However, they are robust treatments and, if you have thin blood vessels or very sensitive skin, you may find an alternative facial treatment more suitable *(see pages 50–55)*. The ideal candidate for steam treatment is someone who has a problem with blackheads or occasional spots and a normal to oily skin type.

1. MAIN PICTURE: Enclose yourself in a towelling 'tent' over the bowl.

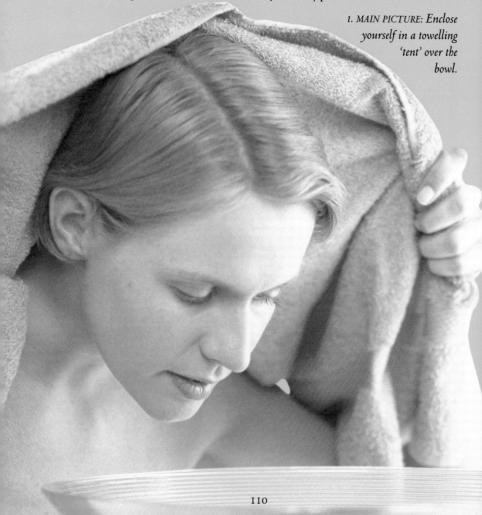

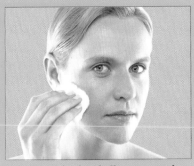

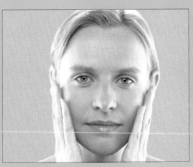

2. Lift your head and allow some of the steam to dry from your face naturally. Then use a gentle toner on cotton wool.

3. When you have removed any dirt, massage in a light day moisturizer — preferably one you have made yourself.

Herbal Steam Bath

6 tablespoons dried mint
1 tablespoon fennel seeds
1 tablespoon dried thyme
1 tablespoon dried marjoram
1 tablespoon lemon juice (optional)
2 litres (8 cups) boiling water

METHOD

Put the dried herbs and lemon juice at the bottom of a large bowl. Pour the boiling water all over them and stir well. Then lean over the bowl and cover your head with a large towel. The steam will open all the pores on your face and help release all the dirt. Stay over the steam bath for 5–10 minutes. Then tone and moisturize your face as usual.

Remember that it is not a good idea to steam your face more than once a week.

EXERCISE AND WASH

11.00 a.m. Put on a comfortable outfit and a pair of trainers or walking shoes and head off for a good walk, maintaining a brisk but comfortable pace. Plan a route that will take you about 30 minutes.

If you have walked at a good pace, you should have got pretty hot and will feel a bit sticky. So back home and time for a shower (or bath). Take a little longer than you did earlier; shampoo your hair and use a conditioner (*see pages 22–7 for home-made ones*).

FINISHING TOUCHES

12.30 p.m. Finally, style your hair, apply your make-up. You will now be ready to take on anything — and all because you took some time just for yourself!

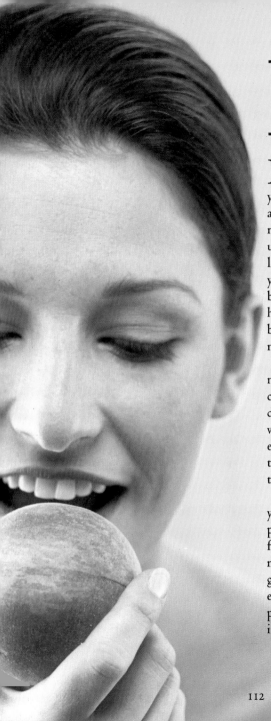

You Are What You Eat

If you have a really special car, household gadget or computer, you read the instruction manual and follow it carefully. Sadly, we do not come with an instruction manual and it is not always easy to follow the correct guidelines. But, if you can get it right, then you will be amazed at the difference a healthy and happy body that is being run on the correct fuel can make to your life and your looks.

To do this you need the right mix of foods and liquids. All the component parts of our bodies depend on the correct supplies of vitamins, minerals and other nutrients to function at their best. Good teeth, hair and nails all begin from the same point – good nutrition.

Vitamin pills are not necessary if you are eating a balanced diet with plenty of variety. However, if you feel you are not getting all the nutrients you should be, then a good-quality multi-vitamin pill each day would be a good insurance policy, until you feel you have improved your diet.

DRINKS

The first and most important ingredient your body needs to work efficiently is water. Whether you choose tap water or mineral water, make sure you have plenty of it. Try to increase your intake to about 1 or 2 litres (2 or 3 pints) a day. It is amazing how much better you will feel, as the water washes away toxins. It is one of the best and most inexpensive treatments for a clear skin and sparkling eyes.

Try to start by drinking just two extra glasses of water each day. If you can then fit in another glass during the evening and perhaps one first thing in the morning, you are already improving your body's input.

TEA AND COFFEE

Both tea and coffee contain caffeine, and tea also contains tannin. Taken in reasonable amounts, neither of them will do you any harm, unless you are particularly susceptible to caffeine. If you think you have a problem with caffeine, then try cutting down on tea and coffee. If you have withdrawal symptoms like headaches and bad temper, then try to kick the habit for a while by drinking herbal teas or just water.

If you are not reliant on caffeine and do not drink more than about four cups every day, then there is no reason you should stop. There has been no scientific research to suggest that limited amounts of tea and coffee are detrimental to health, and a kick-start cup of coffee in the morning may well bring a lot of pleasure to your life. There has even been some research in Japan to suggest that drinking between four and six cups of green tea per day helps prevent cancer. So stay open minded and keep adding in the extra glasses of water.

ALCOHOL

Alcohol is another matter that is so strongly argued in all directions. It is well known that it is a poison and drinking too much is totally inadvisable. However, many studies now agree that regular, but limited, wine drinking can help protect against heart disease. There is also something to be said for its benefits in terms of relaxation and socializing. Stay within safe guidelines of two to three drinks a night and try to have several alcohol-free days in the week to give your liver a rest.

FOOD

There are three basic food groups: proteins, carbohydrates and fats. To run your body correctly, you need to eat all of these things, but in the right proportions. Two thirds of your food should be made up of vegetables, fruit and starchy foods. The other third should comprise low-fat meat, vegetarian proteins and low-fat dairy products. (*See The Healthy Eating Pyramid on pages 116–17.*)

The disappointing thing is that this ideal combination leaves little space for delicious things like chocolate, doughnuts and creamy sauces. The main thing to focus on is the word 'ideal'. There is no need to reach perfection every day. This is the goal to strive for and, providing you reach it more often than not, you are on the road to healthy eating.

As well as allowing your body to function as a whole, the correct mix of nutrients will also nourish your skin, hair and nails to achieve that sparkling-with-health look!

No one can immediately change their diet forever. It takes time, effort and determination to get it right. Take very small steps and you will find you have a better chance of succeeding. Jump in with no preparation, and you will certainly sink!

COMPLEX CARBOHYDRATES

Bread, cereal, rice and pasta should form the main part of your diet. They contain lots of nutrients your body needs for healthy living. Potatoes have vitamin C, wholemeal bread has vitamins B and E, and, more importantly, all these foods provide fibre and easily converted energy. Your body turns all the calories from complex carbohydrates into priority food that it can use immediately. So they give you energy without piling on the weight.

FRUIT AND VEGETABLES

This is another crucial group which very few of us eat enough of. Fruit and vegetables are loaded with goodness, in terms of vitamins, and they help protect the body against everything from viruses and diseases to cancer. They also contain antioxidants to help your body cope with pollutants.

PROTEINS AND DAIRY FOODS

Many people these days eat far too much of this group. The old-fashioned idea of having protein at every meal needs to be reassessed.

However, it is important to have proteins in your diet as these are useful building blocks, which your body uses to help renew cells and build muscle. So look again at the quantities you eat and work out how much you should be eating.

FATS, OILS AND SUGARS

When it comes to these foods, the less the better, particularly on the sugary side. Oils and fats, saturated fat, in particular, are becoming well known for their villainous part in our excess pounds. You do need a certain amount of fat to function properly, but there will usually be enough tied up with the proteins that you eat.

DO YOU NEED TO LOSE WEIGHT?

The main weapons you can use to control your weight are exercise, knowledge of food values and fun. Remember that more important than losing weight is getting fit, and often fitness will stabilize your weight around the correct figure.

If you have a serious weight problem, try joining a slimming organization that uses low-fat, high carbohydrate principles, or team up with a friend who can offer support.

Never strive to be catwalk thin. Life is too short and your health and fitness are too important.

TWO-DAY DETOX DIET

Detox diets are useful occasionally to boost your energy, especially if you have been overindulging, and are feeling lethargic and suffer from cravings. However, they should not be followed any longer than stated, and not while you are working or busy.

DAY ONE

Today you must drink a minimum of 2 litres (4 pints) of water. This will really help your body flush out toxins. The only choice of things to eat today starts and ends with fruit. You can eat more or less as much fruit as you like, but avoid bananas as they are starchy and watery fruits have a much better diuretic effect. Try making fresh fruit salad; pour over some melon juice: it tastes delicious.

DAY TWO

Today you must drink the same amount of water, or more. You can eat any raw fruit and vegetables. Try some fruit additions to salads: mango juice over a green salad tastes wonderful!

THE HEALTHY EATING PYRAMID

THE SUMMIT OF THE PYRAMID

Fats, Oils and Sugars: Sadly, the summit is the smallest section of the pyramid, so, in theory, the one you should eat least of.

THIRD SLICE OF THE PYRAMID

Proteins and Dairy Foods: You should allow about 3–5 portions a day of proteins and dairy products. A portion in this group is about 50–125 g (2–4 oz) lean meat, a small pot of yoghurt, 200 ml (⅓ pint) semi-skimmed or skimmed milk or 300 g (10 oz) cooked beans or lentils.

SECOND SLICE OF THE PYRAMID

Fruit and Vegetables: The ideal would be to aim for 5–8 servings a day, or more if it suits you. To give you an idea of a serving in this group, it would be a piece of fruit or 50–75 g (2–3 oz) of fresh vegetables.

FIRST SLICE OF THE PYRAMID

Complex Carbohydrates (Bread, Cereal, Rice and Pasta): You need to choose at least 6–10 portions from this group each day. To measure roughly how much a portion of these foods might be, allow about one slice (25 g or 1 oz) of wholemeal bread and 1 heaped tablespoon of the pastas and rice (cooked) or 100 g (3½ oz) cooked potatoes.

If you are choosing fats and oils, then try to aim for the polyunsaturated varieties. Olive oil, sunflower oil and avocados are all good sources. Sugar is something most people love and it is hard to wean yourself off it. Try to cut back slowly and it may be easier than you think.

The daily portion here is a lot less than most people eat. The trick with this group is to try to focus on the lower-fat proteins rather than very fatty cuts or burgers and sausages. Chicken and turkey, lean cuts and beans are much better for you.

Try to increase your vegetable intake. Obviously, you should avoid frying your vegetables. Boil them, steam them or roast them without too much added fat. Better still, see how delicious raw vegetables can be. Cereal with fresh fruit is wonderful and fruit with salads transforms them. Try to snack on fruit or vegetables rather than biscuits and chocolate during the day.

Complex carbohydrates are the most important staples, and should form the major part of your diet. They provide high-volume, fibre-filled food that will fill you up without giving you too much fat or sugar.

JUICES

Freshly squeezed fruit and vegetable juices are delicious, and bear no resemblance to the commercially prepared varieties. They enter your bloodstream immediately and give a lovely energy boost. Juicing is a delicious shortcut to consuming some of your necessary fruit and vegetable portions, although some of the fibre is lost in the process. But be careful if you are dieting, as some of these juices use a lot of fruit and therefore contain much natural sugar.

There are various ways to produce juices. The easiest and most effective is to buy a juicer as a separate free-standing machine. Alternatively you can have juice extractor gadget fitted onto an existing food processor or, for some of the juice recipes, a blender or liquidizer can be used. The final option is a traditional lemon squeezer that can be operated by hand and has a strainer to catch pips. This works very well for citrus fruits, but is limited in that it will not process anything else.

Breakfast Nectar

—————— serves I ——————

1–2 oranges
1 apple
1 large carrot

You may have to peel the oranges or squeeze them separately, depending on your juicer. There is no need to peel the apple or the carrot, just give them a really good wash and scrub to remove dirt or chemicals. Juice them both and then add the orange or orange juice. Mix well and pour into a glass over ice. Allow to cool and then enjoy!

Melon Cooler

—————— serves 3–4 ——————

2 oranges
1 large melon (honeydew works well)
pinch powdered ginger (optional)

Squeeze the juice from the oranges and place in the blender. Halve the melon and remove the pips. Using a teaspoon or a melon baller, remove all the melon flesh and place in the blender. Blend rapidly until it is completely smooth. Pour into tall glasses over ice and add the ginger. Allow to cool before drinking.

Carrot, Tomato and Orange Drink

serves 2

1 large orange
4 medium carrots
3 ripe tomatoes (preferably plum tomatoes)
6 sprigs parsley

Squeeze the juice from the orange or peel it and use the juicer. Prepare the carrots and tomatoes to fit into the juicer or blender. Juice the carrots, tomatoes and parsley, then add the orange juice. Pour into glasses over ice. This drink is a good tonic, bursting with vitamin C.

Carrot, Orange and Ginger Juice

serves 1

2 juicy oranges
3 medium carrots
2½ cm (1 in) peeled fresh ginger

Squeeze the juice from the oranges or peel to use the juicer. Juice the carrots and root ginger, then add the orange juice. Pour into a glass over ice – delicious!

Banana Milkshake

serves 2

3 small bananas (as ripe as possible)
300 ml (1¼ cups) skimmed milk
6–8 ice cubes

Peel the bananas and roughly chop them. Place the bananas, milk and ice cubes into a blender and liquidize until it is smooth and frothy. Pour into tall glasses and you will never want to drink a banana milkshake with chemical flavourings ever again. (And this is low calorie!)

Carrot, Pineapple and Cucumber Juice

serves 1–2

2 carrots (medium–large)
1 thick slice pineapple (fresh)
5-cm (2-in) slice cucumber

Prepare the ingredients to fit into the juice extractor and then juice the whole lot together. Pour into a tall glass over ice. This is wonderfully refreshing.

BREAKFAST IDEAS

There are several recipes for a breakfast in a glass that I use frequently. It is important to start the day with something, but not with a heavy, fatty meal like a traditional cooked English breakfast or pancakes with maple syrup and butter stacked up on them! Try the banana milkshake in the Juices section *(see page 118–19)*. It is a wonderful early-morning drink: cold and clean and a good wake-me-up potion! Any of the other juice recipes can also be used for breakfast. The melon drink on a sunny morning is an experience in itself!

Strawberry and Orange Breakfast
serves 1

1 large orange
125 g (4 oz) fresh ripe strawberries
140 g (5 oz) plain bio yoghurt
5 ice cubes

Squeeze the juice from the orange and place in a blender with the strawberries, yoghurt and ice. Whiz until smooth. If it is too thick for you then add some more orange juice or a little skimmed milk.

Fruity Muesli with Yoghurt
serves 3

6 tablespoons crunchy muesli base
250 g (8 oz) (minimum) assorted, chopped, fresh fruit, e.g. grapes, apples, bananas, peaches. (If you are stuck use tinned fruit in juice.)
300 g (10 oz) plain bio yoghurt
3 tablespoons roughly assorted, chopped nuts

Spoon the muesli base into the three bowls, then add a third of the chopped fruit to each bowl. Spoon a third of the yoghurt over each helping and then sprinkle with the nuts.

LUNCHES AND SNACKS

Smoked Mackerel Pâté with Lemon
—————— serves 2 ——————

1 smoked mackerel
125 g (4 oz) low-fat curd-type cheese
a little chopped onion
juice from ½ fresh lemon

Mix all the ingredients in a food processor until completely blended. Place in small pots with a green garnish and serve with pitta bread, bagels, or any other bread you fancy. You can use this recipe for any smoked fish.

Tomato and Kiwi Salad
—————— serves 4 ——————

3 kiwi fruit
6 tomatoes
2 tablespoons pine nuts
45 ml (3 tablespoons) fresh orange juice
5 ml (1 teaspoon) fresh lemon juice

Peel and slice the kiwi fruit and slice the tomatoes. Arrange on a plate with alternate slices of kiwi and tomato. Sprinkle with pine nuts and then mix together the two juices and sprinkle over the salad. Decorate with a sprig of parsley.

Iced Tomato Soup with Basil
—————— serves 6 ——————

1 clove garlic
1 handful fresh basil
10 ml (2 teaspoons) lemon juice
salt and black pepper
300 g (10 oz) low-fat fromage frais
2 x 400-g (14-oz) cans plum tomatoes

Crush the garlic clove with some salt. Place it in a food processor with the basil, lemon juice, lots of pepper and half the fromage frais. Mix well until smooth. Add the tomatoes and blend again. Lastly, add the other half of the fromage frais. Cover and chill until ice cold. Just before serving, check the seasoning and add more salt, pepper, lemon juice, or even a teaspoon of sugar if needed.

MAIN COURSES

Carrot, Date and Pecan Salad
──── serves 4 ────

1 lettuce
450 g (1 lb) new carrots
225 g (8 oz) fresh dates
100 g (4 oz) pecan nut halves
75 ml (5 tablespoons) freshly squeezed
orange juice

Wash lettuce well and use the leaves to make a base for the salad on a serving dish. Peel, top and tail the carrots, then chop into matchstick-sized pieces. Remove the stones and skins from the dates and chop into quarters. Mix together the carrots, dates and nuts, add the orange juice and stir well. Heap the salad over the lettuce leaves and serve immediately or chill in the fridge until required. This will keep in the fridge for several hours, but not overnight. You may also like to try using walnuts, hazelnuts or almonds instead of pecans.

Salmon Steaks in Silver Foil
──── serves 4 ────

4 salmon steaks
60 ml (4 tablespoons) fresh orange juice
1 handful fresh parsley
1 bunch fresh chives
1 small bunch fresh mint
60 ml (4 tablespoons) fresh lemon juice
watercress to garnish

Place each salmon steak in the centre of a piece of foil. Add 1 tablespoon of orange juice and a few sprigs of each herb to each parcel. Wrap the parcels loosely so that they are sealed but baggy. Place in the oven (pre-heated to 170°C, 350°F or Gas Mark 4) for about 15 minutes. When cooked allow them to stand and, when serving, remove the herbs and pour 1 tablespoon of lemon juice over each steak and garnish with watercress. Serve with seasonal vegetables and a salad.

Tuna and Rice Salad
serves 3

175 g (¾ cup) uncooked long-grain rice
3 tomatoes
4 spring onions
2 tablespoons chopped fresh herbs
1 ripe mango
2–3 handfuls chopped fresh salad leaves
200-g (7-oz) can tuna in brine
3 hard-boiled eggs

DRESSING

juice from 1 lime
10 ml (2 teaspoons) balsamic vinegar
1 garlic clove, finely chopped
1 teaspoon ground cumin
45 ml (3 tablespoons) fresh orange juice
45 ml (3 tablespoons) olive oil
salt and freshly ground black pepper

Mix together all the dressing ingredients except the oil. Then whisk in the oil and leave to stand.

Cook the rice and leave to cool. Chop the tomatoes, spring onions and herbs; peel and chop the mango. Add to the cooled rice. Whisk the dressing again, pour over the rice mixture and combine well.

Divide the salad leaves between the plates and pile some rice mixture in the centre. Drain the tuna, and shell and quarter the hard-boiled eggs. Arrange the tuna and eggs on top of the rice.

Lemon Chicken with Cashew Nuts
serves 4

2 large chicken breasts
1 clove garlic
2½ cm (1 in) peeled fresh ginger
1 fresh lemon
45 ml (3 tablespoons) soya sauce
75 ml (5 tablespoons) water
30 ml (2 tablespoons) sherry
1 tablespoon cornflour or cornstarch
15 ml (1 tablespoon) oil to stir-fry
125 g (4 oz) cashew nuts

Cut the chicken breasts into thin strips and place in a bowl. Crush the garlic, finely chop the ginger, and mix them into the chicken. Using a zester, remove all the zest from the lemon skin and add to the chicken. Then squeeze the juice from the lemon and put to one side. Place the soya sauce, water and sherry in a small bowl and add the cornflour to make a thin paste.

Heat up a well-seasoned wok and add the oil. Cook the chicken mixture in the wok rapidly for 5–10 minutes, turning occasionally. Stir in the cornflour mixture, turning the chicken constantly. When the chicken is almost cooked, add the lemon juice and cashew nuts, and cook for a couple more minutes. If the mixture is becoming dry, add a little more water. Serve with boiled rice and Chinese vegetables.

DESSERTS

Peach Brûlée
—— serves 2 ——

*2 fresh peaches (tinned in juice are fine if
you cannot get fresh)
150 g (5 oz) low-fat fromage frais
2 tablespoons brown demerara sugar*

Peel the peaches (if they are fresh)
and slice them into small chunks so
they are easy to eat. Divide the fruit
between two heatproof containers.
Cover this layer of peaches with the
fromage frais and make it fairly
smooth on top. Sprinkle a tablespoon of sugar over each container.
Heat the grill to its hottest setting
and, watching all the time, grill
until the sugar has all melted and
bubbles form on the surface.
Remove from the heat and allow to cool. This pud-
ding is delicious chilled in the
fridge for a couple of hours before
serving.

Instant Banana Ice Cream
—— serves 2 ——

*3 chopped bananas (frozen for at least
4 hours)
45 ml (3 tablespoons) fromage frais
skimmed milk as necessary*

Most fruits respond to this instant
recipe (ready-frozen strawberries,
raspberries, mango, pineapple,
whatever you choose). It is important to make sure the fruit is completely frozen as this adds body to
the ice cream.

Place the frozen bananas in a
food processor and add the fromage
frais. Process until it makes a
smooth ice cream. If it sticks or
seems too lumpy, cautiously
add a spoonful of skimmed
milk at a time until it

loosens up a bit. Beware of adding too much milk as this turns it into an equally delicious fruit fool, not an ice cream. Serve in bowls garnished with mint leaves or a fresh strawberry.

Mango Heaven
serves 2

2 ripe mangos
300 g (10 oz) plain bio yoghurt
150 g (5 oz) low-fat curd-type cheese
25 g (1 oz) flaked almonds

Peel the mangos and remove as much of the flesh as possible. Combine the mango flesh, yoghurt and cheese in a food processor, until smooth. Then pour into pretty sundae glasses and decorate with the flaked almonds.

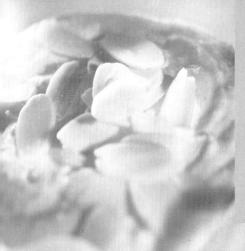

IMPROVE YOUR HEALTH

Food, exercise, relaxation and beauty care are each important to your overall health. So try to persuade yourself into a healthier lifestyle. But never ask too much; encourage and cajole yourself as though you were dealing with a difficult child and maybe you will win through. All methods are available and acceptable. Try bribing yourself, for example: If I follow my health plan for a week, I will buy that new jumper. Or if you have shorter horizons, then try: If I get through the whole of today with no chocolate then I will treat myself to a new lipstick or to a special beauty treatment.

Go for your personal health, but go slowly. Every journey, no matter how long, starts with a single step, and any step that lasts is a triumph. With every improvement you make, see your natural beauty radiate.

Good luck!

BIBLIOGRAPHY

Aromatherapy, Judith Jackson, London: Dorling Kindersley, 1987

The Aromatherapy Kit, Charla Devereux, Boston: Charles E. Tuttle Co., Inc., 1993; London: Headline, 1993

The Complete New Herbal, Richard Mabey, London: Elm Tree Books, 1988

Culpeper's Colour Herbal, New York: Sterling Publishing Co., Inc., 1992; Berkshire: W. Foulsham, 1983

The Encyclopaedia of Essential Oils, J. Lawless, Dorset: Element, 1992

The Fragrant Pharmacy, V. A. Worwood, London: Bantam, 1994

Gerard's Herbal, London: Studio Editions, 1985

The Green Witch, Barbara Griggs, Rochester, VT: Inner Traditions, 1994; London: Vermilion, 1993

Herbal Delights, Mrs. C. F. Leyel, New York: Random House Value Publishing, 1986; London: Faber and Faber, 1937

Herbal Health and Beauty Book, H. Boddie, Pomfret, VT: Trafalgar Square, 1996; London: Optima, 1994

The Magic of Herbs, David Conway, Devon: Reader's Union, 1976

Making Your Own Cosmetics, James Sholto Douglas, London: Pelham Books, 1979

The Story of Lavender, S. Festing, Sutton: Heritage in Sutton Leisure, 1989

Three by Szekely (Vitamins, Minerals and Herbs), E. B. Szekely, Connecticut: Keats Publishing Inc., 1983

USEFUL ADDRESSES

Please enclose a stamped addressed envelope for catalogues.

UNITED KINGDOM

Neal's Yard Remedies, 15 Neal's Yard, Covent Garden, London WC2H 9DP Tel: 0171 379 7222, mail orders: 0161 8317875. And 3 Golden Cross, Cornmarket, Oxford OXI 3EU Tel: 01865 245436
They sell a huge range of ingredients including beeswax granules, base oils, essential oils and flower waters.

G. Baldwin and Company, 173 Walworth Road, London SE17 IRW Tel: 0171 703 5550
Very wide range of herbs and roots, barks and powders. They also stock beeswax and cocoa butter, floral waters and oils.

The Tisserand Institute, 63 Church Road, Hove, Sussex BN3 2BD Tel: 01273 206640
Good range of all supplies needed for aromatherapy – full selection of essential oils.

UNITED STATES

The organizations below are suppliers of essential oils and information.

The American Society for Phytotherapy and Aromatherapy International Inc., PO Box 3679, South Pasadena, California 91031
Tel: 818 457 1742

Aroma Vera Inc, 5901 Rodeo Road, Los Angeles, CA 90016
Tel: 800 669 9514

International Federation of Aromatherapists, c/o Allison Russell, 35 Bydown Street, Neutral Bay, NSW 2089
Tel: 01 902 240125

Essential Therapeutics, 58 Easey Street, Collingwood, Victoria 3066
Tel: 03 419 7711

Bronson & Jacobs Pty Ltd., Parkview Drive, Australia Centre, Homebush NSW 2140
Tel: 02 394 3288

AUSTRALIA

The organizations below are suppliers of essential oils and information.

INDEX

ACKNOWLEDGEMENTS

There are so many people to thank as there was so much work involved in putting all these recipes together. My first thanks must go to my family – especially my husband Adrian for taking so many responsibilities away from me so that I could meet all the deadlines. Also my thanks to Ian Jackson for letting me take on the project and for all the help from Zoë Hughes and Sophie Bevan as my brilliant editors. Thank you also to all those of you who tested the products for me and let me use your suggestions.

EDDISON•SADD EDITIONS

Editor	Sophie Bevan
Proofreader	Michele Turney
Indexer	Dorothy Frame
Senior Art Editor	Sarah Howerd
Photographers	Stephen Marwood and David Kelly
Make-up Artist	Lynn Jackett
Models	Sandra, Gail and Shriti
Production	Hazel Kirkman and Charles James

Eddison Sadd would like to thank Neal's Yard Remedies, London, for donating all the dried herbs and basic ingredients for the photography.